ASTHMA AND DIET

A Science-Based Guide to Managing Symptoms through Nutrition

DR. RACHEL H. HARRISON

COPYRIGHT © 2024 by Dr. Rachel H. Harrison

TABLE OF CONTENTS

INTRODUCTION

Welcome to 'Asthma and Diet', your comprehensive guide to understanding and managing asthma through informed dietary choices and lifestyle modifications. As a chronic respiratory condition, asthma significantly impacts daily life. While medication is crucial, research highlights the importance of diet in managing symptoms and promoting overall well-being.

This book empowers you with knowledge and tools to make informed decisions about your diet and lifestyle, enabling proactive steps to reduce inflammation, avoid triggers, and enhance quality of life. The following chapters provide in-depth information on asthma, including types, symptoms, causes, and triggers, alongside the scientific connection between nutrition and respiratory health. Practical advice on meal planning, grocery shopping, and cooking asthma-friendly recipes is also included, plus guidance on lifestyle factors like exercise, stress management, and creating a supportive home environment.

Personal stories and expert advice are woven throughout, making this handbook an invaluable resource for anyone seeking to manage asthma and improve overall health through nutrition and lifestyle changes.

CHAPTER 1

30 fascinating facts about Asthma

1. Chronic Condition: Asthma is a chronic respiratory condition that affects the airways in the lungs, causing them to become inflamed and narrow.

2. Symptoms: Common symptoms include wheezing, shortness of breath, chest tightness, and coughing, especially at night or early in the morning.

3. Triggers: Asthma attacks can be triggered by allergens (pollen, dust mites, pet dander), irritants (smoke, pollution), respiratory infections, exercise, and stress.

4. Prevalence: Asthma affects approximately 300 million people worldwide.

5. Childhood Onset: Asthma often starts in childhood, but it can develop at any age.

6. Genetics: Genetics play a significant role in the development of asthma; having a family history of asthma or allergies increases the risk.

7. Environmental Factors: Exposure to pollutants and allergens in the environment can increase the risk of developing asthma.

8. Exercise-Induced Asthma: Physical activity can trigger asthma symptoms, a condition known as exercise-induced bronchoconstriction (EIB).

9. Occupational Asthma: Certain occupations expose individuals to irritants that can cause asthma, such as chemicals, dust, and fumes.

10. No Cure: There is currently no cure for asthma, but it can be managed effectively with proper treatment and lifestyle changes.

11. Medications: Asthma medications are typically divided into two categories: long-term control medications (inhaled corticosteroids) and quick-relief medications (bronchodilators).

12. Inhalers: Inhalers are the most common device for delivering asthma medication directly to the lungs.

13. Asthma Action Plan: An asthma action plan, created with a healthcare provider, helps individuals manage their condition and recognize early signs of an attack.

14. Allergy Testing: Allergy testing can help identify specific triggers and guide treatment.

15. Asthma Control Test (ACT): The ACT is a simple questionnaire that helps individuals and healthcare providers assess asthma control.

16. Peak Flow Meter: A peak flow meter is a device used to measure how well air is moving out of the lungs, helping to monitor asthma.

17. Impact on Daily Life: Without proper management, asthma can significantly impact daily activities and quality of life.

18. Emergency Situations: Severe asthma attacks can be life-threatening and require immediate medical attention.

19. Weather Influence: Cold air, changes in weather, and humidity can exacerbate asthma symptoms.

20. Secondhand Smoke: Exposure to secondhand smoke is a significant risk factor for asthma, especially in children.

21. Respiratory Infections: Colds and other respiratory infections can worsen asthma symptoms.

22. Asthma and Pregnancy: Pregnant women with asthma need to manage their condition carefully to ensure the health of both mother and baby.

23. Diet and Asthma: Some studies suggest that a diet rich in fruits, vegetables, and omega-3 fatty acids may help reduce asthma symptoms.

24. Obesity Link: Obesity is a risk factor for developing asthma and can make symptoms worse.

25. Asthma Education: Education about asthma self-management is crucial for controlling the condition and preventing attacks.

26. Impact on Sleep: Asthma symptoms often worsen at night, leading to sleep disturbances and fatigue.

27. Childhood Asthma Management: Proper management of childhood asthma is essential for normal growth and development.

28. Importance of Adherence: Adhering to prescribed medication regimens is crucial for keeping asthma under control.

29. Asthma and Mental Health: Chronic asthma can impact mental health, leading to anxiety and depression.

30. Regular Check-ups: Regular check-ups with a healthcare provider are important to monitor asthma control and adjust treatment as necessary.

These facts provide a comprehensive overview of asthma, its impact, and the importance of effective management.

CHAPTER 2

Welcome to the Asthma and Diet

Asthma is a chronic respiratory condition that affects millions of people worldwide, causing symptoms such as wheezing, shortness of breath, chest tightness, and coughing. While there is no cure for asthma, effective management strategies can significantly improve the quality of life for those affected. One of the most impactful yet often overlooked strategies is diet. This book, "Asthma and Diet," is dedicated to exploring the crucial role that diet plays in managing asthma and providing practical guidance on how to make dietary choices that support respiratory health.

Purpose and Goals

The primary purpose of the "Asthma and Diet" is to empower individuals with asthma and their caregivers with the knowledge and tools necessary to manage asthma symptoms through dietary interventions.

The goals of this book include:

1. Educating Readers on Asthma: Providing a thorough understanding of what asthma is, its causes, and how it affects the body. This foundational knowledge is essential for understanding the role of diet in managing the condition.

2. Highlighting the Connection Between Diet and Asthma: Presenting evidence-based research and scientific studies that demonstrate how certain foods and nutrients can influence asthma symptoms and overall lung function.

3. Identifying Asthma Triggers in Food: Helping readers recognize foods and food additives that can trigger asthma symptoms, allowing them to make informed choices about what to avoid in their diets.

4. Promoting Asthma-Friendly Foods: Introducing foods that have been shown to support respiratory health, reduce inflammation, and boost the immune system. Emphasis will be placed on incorporating these foods into daily meals.

5. Providing Practical Meal Planning and Recipes: Offering a variety of delicious and nutritious recipes that are tailored to the needs of asthma patients. These recipes are designed to be easy to prepare and include asthma-friendly ingredients.

6. Supporting Lifestyle Changes: Discussing other lifestyle factors that can impact asthma, such as exercise, stress management, and environmental factors. This holistic approach ensures that all aspects of asthma management are addressed.

7. Sharing Personal Stories and Expert Advice: Including real-life stories from individuals who have successfully managed their asthma through diet and lifestyle changes,

as well as expert tips from nutritionists and medical professionals.

How to Use This Book

The "Asthma and Diet" is designed to be a practical and user-friendly guide.

Here are some tips on how to make the most of this book:

1. Start with the Basics: Begin by reading the sections on understanding asthma and the role of diet in asthma management. This foundational knowledge will help you appreciate the importance of dietary choices in managing your condition.

2. Identify Your Triggers: Use the chapters on foods that may trigger asthma to identify any potential dietary triggers in your current eating habits. This will help you make informed decisions about what to avoid.

3. Incorporate Asthma-Friendly Foods: Explore the chapters on essential nutrients and foods to include in your diet. Start incorporating these foods into your meals to support your respiratory health.

4. Plan Your Meals: Utilize the meal planning tips and sample meal plans provided in the book. These plans are designed to make it easier for you to create balanced, nutritious, and asthma-friendly meals.

5. Try the Recipes: Experiment with the breakfast, lunch, dinner, and snack recipes included in the book. These recipes are not only delicious but also specifically designed to help manage asthma symptoms.

6. Adopt a Holistic Approach: Read the sections on exercise, stress management, and environmental factors to understand how these lifestyle elements can affect your asthma. Incorporate the tips provided to create a comprehensive asthma management plan.

7. Stay Informed and Inspired: Benefit from the personal stories and expert advice included in the book. These stories can provide motivation and insight into how others have successfully managed their asthma through diet and lifestyle changes.

8. Use the Appendices as a Reference: The glossary of terms, frequently asked questions, and index are valuable resources for quick reference. Use them to clarify concepts and find specific information easily.

9. Personalize Your Approach: Everyone's experience with asthma is unique. Use the information and tips provided in the book to create a personalized asthma management plan that works best for you. Consult with healthcare providers to tailor the advice to your specific needs.

The "Asthma and Diet" is more than just a cookbook; it is a comprehensive guide to understanding and managing asthma through diet and lifestyle. By following the guidance provided in this book, you can take proactive steps towards improving your respiratory health and enhancing your overall quality of life. Welcome to your journey towards better asthma management through the power of diet!

Who This Book Is For?

The "Asthma and Diet" is intended for a diverse audience, recognizing that asthma affects individuals across various demographics and life stages. This book is designed to be a comprehensive resource for anyone seeking to improve their asthma management through dietary and lifestyle changes.

Here's a closer look at who will benefit from this handbook:

Individuals with Asthma

1. Newly Diagnosed Patients:

• Understanding the Condition: Individuals who have recently been diagnosed with asthma will find this book invaluable for understanding the basics of the condition, its causes, and how it affects their daily lives.

• Early Dietary Interventions: Early-stage patients can learn about dietary changes that can prevent the progression of symptoms and improve their quality of life from the onset.

2. Long-term Asthma Patients:

• Enhancing Management: Those who have been living with asthma for a longer time can discover new strategies and dietary adjustments to further enhance their asthma management.

• Breaking Plateaus: For patients whose asthma management has plateaued, this book provides fresh insights and approaches to overcome challenges and improve lung function.

3. Children and Adolescents with Asthma:

• Parental Guidance: Parents of children and adolescents with asthma will find practical advice on preparing asthma-friendly meals that cater to young pilates while ensuring nutritional adequacy.

• Empowering Young Patients: Older children and teens can learn to make informed food choices independently, fostering a proactive approach to their health.

Caregivers and Family Members

1. Primary Caregivers:

• Meal Preparation: Caregivers who prepare meals for individuals with asthma will benefit from understanding which foods to include and avoid, and how to create balanced, nutritious meals.

• Holistic Care: In addition to dietary guidance, caregivers can learn about other lifestyle adjustments that can support the overall well-being of their loved ones.

2. Supportive Family Members:

• Creating a Supportive Environment: Family members can play a significant role in managing asthma by understanding dietary triggers and ensuring the home environment is conducive to respiratory health.

• Shared Meals and Habits: This book encourages family-wide adoption of asthma-friendly diets, promoting healthier eating habits for everyone.

Health and Wellness Professionals

1. Nutritionists and Dietitians:

• Evidence-Based Guidance: Nutritionists and dietitians can use this book as a resource to provide evidence-based dietary advice to their clients with asthma.

• Customizing Diet Plans: The detailed information on nutrients, foods, and meal planning can aid professionals in creating customized diet plans tailored to individual needs.

2. Healthcare Providers:

• Complementary Management: Doctors, respiratory therapists, and other healthcare providers can recommend this book as part of a comprehensive asthma management plan, complementing medical treatments with dietary and lifestyle changes.

• Patient Education: The book can serve as an educational tool to help patients understand the importance of diet in managing asthma.

Individuals Interested in Respiratory Health

1. Health Enthusiasts:

• Preventive Measures: People who are interested in maintaining optimal respiratory health, even if they do not have asthma, can benefit from the dietary principles outlined in this book.

• Holistic Wellness: The book's focus on a holistic approach to health, including stress management and exercise, appeals to those pursuing overall wellness.

2. Those at Risk of Developing Asthma:

• Proactive Steps: Individuals with a family history of asthma or other risk factors can use the dietary and lifestyle recommendations in this book to potentially reduce their risk of developing asthma or mitigate its severity.

Educational Institutions and Community Programs

1. Schools and Colleges:

• Health Education: Schools and colleges can incorporate the book's content into health education curricula, teaching students about the impact of diet on asthma and general health.

• Support for Students: Educational institutions can provide resources to students with asthma, helping them manage their condition effectively.

2. Community Health Programs:

• Public Health Initiatives: Community health programs aimed at improving respiratory health can use this book as part of their outreach and educational efforts.

• Workshops and Seminars: The book's content can be used to design workshops and seminars focused on asthma management through diet and lifestyle.

The "Asthma and Diet" is a valuable resource for a wide audience, from individuals with asthma and their caregivers to health professionals and wellness enthusiasts. By offering comprehensive, evidence-based information and practical guidance, this book aims to empower readers to take control of their asthma management through informed dietary and lifestyle choices. No matter who you are, if you are interested in improving respiratory health, this handbook is for you.

CHAPTER 3

Understanding Asthma

What is Asthma?

Asthma is a chronic respiratory condition characterized by inflammation and narrowing of the airways, leading to difficulty in breathing. This condition affects millions of people worldwide and can range from mild to severe. Understanding asthma involves recognizing its symptoms, triggers, and the mechanisms behind its manifestation.

Asthma primarily affects the bronchial tubes, which are the airways that carry air in and out of the lungs. When these airways become inflamed, they swell and produce extra mucus, causing the muscles around them to tighten. This combination of factors leads to the hallmark symptoms of asthma: wheezing, shortness of breath, chest tightness, and coughing. These symptoms can vary in intensity and frequency, often becoming worse during physical activity or at night.

Definition and Overview

Asthma is defined as a chronic inflammatory disease of the airways, marked by recurring episodes of wheezing, breathlessness, chest tightness, and coughing. The condition is typically reversible, either spontaneously or with treatment, although it can lead to persistent changes in the airway structure over time.

Key Characteristics of Asthma:

1. Chronic Inflammation: The underlying issue in asthma is chronic inflammation of the airways. This inflammation makes the airways hyperresponsive to various triggers, leading to swelling and narrowing that impede airflow.

2. Airway Hyperresponsiveness: Individuals with asthma have airways that are overly sensitive to a variety of stimuli, including allergens, pollutants, cold air, exercise,

and respiratory infections. These triggers can cause the airways to constrict more than they would in non-asthmatic individuals.

3. Reversible Airflow Obstruction: Unlike other chronic lung diseases, the airway obstruction in asthma is generally reversible. This means that with proper treatment, the airways can return to normal functioning, though this reversibility may decrease with chronic, poorly managed asthma.

Asthma Symptoms:

• Wheezing: A high-pitched whistling sound made while breathing, particularly during exhalation.

• Shortness of Breath: Difficulty in breathing or a feeling of breathlessness.

• Chest Tightness: A sensation of constriction or pressure in the chest.

• Coughing: Often worse at night or early in the morning, coughing can be a persistent symptom that disrupts sleep and daily activities.

Common Triggers of Asthma:

1. Allergens: Dust mites, pollen, pet dander, mold, and other allergens can trigger asthma symptoms.

2. Irritants: Tobacco smoke, pollution, strong odors, and chemical fumes can exacerbate asthma.

3. Exercise: Physical activity, especially in cold air, can induce exercise-induced bronchoconstriction.

4. Respiratory Infections: Colds, flu, and other respiratory infections can worsen asthma symptoms.

5. Weather: Cold air, changes in weather, and high humidity levels can trigger asthma.

6. Emotional Stress: Strong emotions and stress can lead to hyperventilation and trigger asthma symptoms.

Mechanisms Behind Asthma:

• Inflammation: Persistent inflammation in the bronchial tubes leads to swelling and mucus production, reducing the airway diameter.

• Bronchoconstriction: The muscles surrounding the airways tighten, further narrowing the airways and making it difficult to breathe.

• Mucus Production: Increased mucus secretion clogs the airways, exacerbating the difficulty in breathing.

Asthma Diagnosis and Management:

Diagnosing asthma typically involves a combination of medical history, physical examination, and lung function tests. Spirometry is a common test used to measure how much air one can inhale and exhale, and how quickly one can exhale. Additional tests may include allergy testing and imaging studies.

Treatment Options:

1. Medications:

• Quick-Relief Medications: Also known as rescue inhalers, these medications (e.g., short-acting beta agonists) provide immediate relief from asthma symptoms.

• Long-Term Control Medications: These include inhaled corticosteroids, long-acting beta agonists, leukotriene modifiers, and other medications designed to control chronic symptoms and prevent attacks.

2. Lifestyle Adjustments:

• Avoiding Triggers: Identifying and avoiding known asthma triggers is crucial in managing the condition.

• Healthy Diet and Exercise: Maintaining a healthy diet and regular exercise routine can improve overall lung function and reduce asthma symptoms.

• Stress Management: Techniques such as meditation, yoga, and deep-breathing exercises can help manage stress and reduce asthma flare-ups.

3. Monitoring and Regular Check-Ups:

• Asthma Action Plan: Developing a personalized asthma action plan with a healthcare provider can help manage symptoms and respond appropriately to asthma attacks.

• Regular Medical Reviews: Regular check-ups with a healthcare provider ensure that asthma is being managed effectively and that treatment plans are adjusted as needed.

Understanding asthma is the first step in effectively managing the condition. By recognizing its symptoms, identifying triggers, and following a comprehensive management plan, individuals with asthma can lead healthy, active lives. This book aims to provide the knowledge and tools necessary to achieve optimal asthma control through informed dietary and lifestyle choices.

CHAPTER 4

Types of Asthma

Asthma is a heterogeneous disease with various types, each having distinct characteristics, triggers, and treatment approaches. Recognizing the different types of asthma can help in tailoring management strategies to effectively control symptoms and improve quality of life.

1. Allergic (Extrinsic) Asthma

Definition: Allergic asthma, also known as extrinsic asthma, is the most common type of asthma. It is triggered by exposure to allergens such as pollen, dust mites, pet dander, mold, and certain foods.

Characteristics:

• Often associated with other allergic conditions like allergic rhinitis (hay fever) and eczema.

• Commonly begins in childhood but can occur at any age.

• Symptoms are often seasonal or related to specific environmental exposures.

Management:

• Identifying and avoiding allergens is crucial.

• Medications may include inhaled corticosteroids, antihistamines, and leukotriene modifiers.

• Allergen immunotherapy (allergy shots) may be considered in severe cases.

2. Non-Allergic (Intrinsic) Asthma

Definition: Non-allergic asthma, also known as intrinsic asthma, is not triggered by allergens. Instead, it is often triggered by factors such as stress, exercise, cold air, smoke, or respiratory infections.

Characteristics:

• More common in adults, especially women.

• Symptoms can occur year-round and are not linked to allergic reactions.

• Often more severe and difficult to control than allergic asthma.

Management:

• Avoiding triggers such as smoke, strong odors, and cold air is important.

• Medications may include inhaled corticosteroids, bronchodilators, and other long-term control medications.

• Stress management techniques and regular exercise can help in symptom management.

3. Exercise-Induced Asthma (EIA)

Definition: Exercise-induced asthma, or exercise-induced bronchoconstriction (EIB), is triggered by physical activity. Symptoms typically appear during or after exercise.

Characteristics:

• Symptoms include coughing, wheezing, shortness of breath, and chest tightness during or after exercise.

• Common in both children and adults, particularly athletes.

Management:
• Warming up before exercise and cooling down after can help reduce symptoms.
• Using quick-relief inhalers (short-acting beta-agonists) before exercise.
• Regular use of long-term control medications may be necessary for frequent exercisers.

4. Occupational Asthma

Definition: Occupational asthma is caused by exposure to irritants in the workplace, such as chemicals, dust, gasses, or fumes.

Characteristics:
• Symptoms improve when away from the workplace and worsen upon returning.
• Common in industries like manufacturing, farming, hairdressing, and healthcare.

Management:

• Identifying and minimizing exposure to workplace irritants is crucial.

• Personal protective equipment (PPE) may be necessary.

• Medications include inhaled corticosteroids and bronchodilators.

5. Nocturnal Asthma

Definition: Nocturnal asthma refers to asthma symptoms that worsen at night, disrupting sleep.

Characteristics:

• Symptoms include coughing, wheezing, and breathlessness during the night.

• Can be linked to factors such as allergens in the bedroom, cooler night air, or the body's natural circadian rhythms.

Management:

• Keeping the sleeping environment free of allergens (e.g., using hypoallergenic bedding).

- Ensuring proper use of asthma medications, particularly before bedtime.
- Using long-acting bronchodilators or inhaled corticosteroids.

6. Aspirin-Induced Asthma (AIA)

Definition: Aspirin-induced asthma, also known as aspirin-exacerbated respiratory disease (AERD), is triggered by the ingestion of aspirin or other non-steroidal anti-inflammatory drugs (NSAIDs).

Characteristics:

- Symptoms include severe asthma attacks, nasal congestion, and sinusitis after taking aspirin or NSAIDs.
- Often associated with nasal polyps.

Management:

- Avoiding aspirin and NSAIDs is essential.
- Using alternative pain relievers, such as acetaminophen, under medical guidance.
- Medications include inhaled corticosteroids, leukotriene modifiers, and nasal corticosteroids.

7. Cough-Variant Asthma

Definition: Cough-variant asthma is characterized primarily by a persistent cough rather than the typical asthma symptoms of wheezing and breathlessness.

Characteristics:

• Chronic cough that does not respond to typical cough medications.

• Often misdiagnosed as chronic bronchitis or postnasal drip.

Management:

• Diagnosing via lung function tests and response to asthma medications.

• Treating with inhaled corticosteroids and bronchodilators.

Common Symptoms

Asthma symptoms can vary widely among individuals and may fluctuate over time. Recognizing these symptoms is crucial for effective management and timely intervention.

1. Wheezing

Description: Wheezing is a high-pitched whistling sound produced during breathing, particularly during exhalation.

Causes:

• Airway constriction due to inflammation and mucus buildup.

• Common in both acute asthma attacks and chronic asthma.

2. Shortness of Breath

Description: Shortness of breath, or dyspnea, is a sensation of difficulty in breathing or feeling breathless.

Causes:

• Narrowed airways restrict airflow, making it hard to breathe deeply.

• Often exacerbated by physical exertion, stress, or exposure to triggers.

3. Chest Tightness

Description: Chest tightness is a sensation of constriction or pressure in the chest.

Causes:

• Muscle tightening around the airways.

• Inflammation and mucus production contribute to this feeling.

4. Coughing

Description: Persistent coughing, especially at night or early in the morning, is a common asthma symptom.

Causes:

• Airway irritation and mucus buildup.

• Can be the primary symptom in cough-variant asthma.

5. Difficulty Sleeping

Description: Asthma symptoms often worsen at night, leading to difficulty falling asleep or frequent awakenings.

Causes:

• Increased exposure to allergens in the bedroom.
• Natural nighttime decrease in airway function.

6. Rapid Breathing

Description: Rapid breathing, or tachypnea, is an increased rate of breathing.

Causes:

• The body's response to decreased oxygen levels due to airway obstruction.
• Often accompanies severe asthma attacks.

7. Anxiety or Panic

Description: Anxiety or panic can result from the sensation of not being able to breathe properly.

Causes:

• The psychological impact of breathlessness and wheezing.

• Can exacerbate asthma symptoms, creating a cycle of stress and respiratory distress.

Understanding the different types of asthma and recognizing common symptoms are essential steps in managing this chronic condition. Effective management involves avoiding triggers, adhering to prescribed medications, and maintaining a healthy lifestyle. This comprehensive approach can significantly improve the quality of life for individuals with asthma.

CHAPTER 5

Causes and Triggers of Asthma

Asthma is a complex condition influenced by a variety of factors, including genetic predisposition, environmental exposures, and lifestyle choices. Understanding the causes and triggers of asthma can help individuals manage their condition more effectively and reduce the frequency and severity of asthma attacks.

Environmental Factors

Environmental factors play a significant role in the onset and exacerbation of asthma symptoms. These factors can vary widely depending on geographical location, season, and individual sensitivities.

Here, we explore the primary environmental triggers that can contribute to asthma:

1. Allergens: Allergens are substances that can cause an allergic reaction and are a common trigger for asthma. **Common allergens include:**

• Pollen: Seasonal pollen from trees, grasses, and weeds can trigger asthma symptoms in sensitive individuals. This type of asthma is often referred to as seasonal allergic asthma.

• Dust Mites: These microscopic creatures live in household dust and are a common indoor allergen. They thrive in bedding, upholstery, and carpets.

• Pet Dander: Proteins found in the skin flakes, urine, and saliva of pets like cats and dogs can trigger asthma.

• Mold: Indoor and outdoor molds produce spores that can be inhaled and trigger asthma symptoms. Mold thrives in damp, humid environments.

• Cockroach Droppings: The feces, saliva, and body parts of cockroaches can trigger asthma, especially in urban areas where cockroach infestations are more common.

2. Air Pollutants: Air pollution is a major environmental factor that can exacerbate asthma symptoms.

Common air pollutants include:

• Outdoor Air Pollution: Emissions from vehicles, industrial facilities, and power plants release pollutants like ozone, nitrogen dioxide, and particulate matter that can irritate the airways.

• Indoor Air Pollution: Sources of indoor pollution include tobacco smoke, wood-burning stoves, gas stoves, and volatile organic compounds (VOCs) from household products and building materials.

3. Tobacco Smoke: Tobacco smoke is a potent asthma trigger. Both active smoking and exposure to secondhand smoke can cause significant respiratory irritation and inflammation. Smoking during pregnancy can also increase the risk of the child developing asthma.

4. Weather Conditions: Weather conditions can influence asthma symptoms. Specific weather-related triggers include:

• Cold Air: Breathing in cold, dry air can cause the airways to constrict, leading to asthma symptoms.

• Hot, Humid Air: High humidity levels can increase the presence of mold and dust mites, which can trigger asthma. Hot, humid air can also make breathing more difficult.

• Sudden Temperature Changes: Rapid changes in temperature can irritate the airways and trigger asthma attacks.

5. Respiratory Infections: Respiratory infections such as the common cold, influenza, and bronchitis can exacerbate asthma symptoms. These infections can cause increased inflammation and mucus production in the airways.

6. Occupational Exposures: Occupational asthma is triggered by exposure to irritants in the workplace. **Common occupational triggers include:**

• Chemical Fumes: Exposure to chemicals such as solvents, cleaning agents, and pesticides can irritate the airways.

• Dust: Industrial dust from construction, woodworking, and mining can trigger asthma.

• Gasses and Vapors: Gasses like ammonia, chlorine, and sulfur dioxide are common in certain industries and can cause respiratory irritation.

7.   Physical   Activity: Exercise-induced bronchoconstriction (EIB), also known as exercise-induced asthma, occurs when physical activity triggers asthma symptoms. This is often due to breathing in dry, cold air during exercise, which can irritate the airways.

8. Emotional Stress: Emotional stress and strong emotions such as anxiety, anger, and laughter can trigger asthma symptoms. Stress can lead to hyperventilation and increased airway reactivity, making asthma worse.

9. Food and Additives: Certain foods and food additives can trigger asthma symptoms in some individuals.

These include:

• Sulfites: Preservatives found in foods and drinks like dried fruits, wine, and processed foods can trigger asthma.

• Food Allergies: Common food allergens such as nuts, shellfish, and eggs can cause allergic reactions and trigger asthma symptoms.

Environmental factors are significant contributors to asthma exacerbations. By identifying and avoiding specific triggers, individuals with asthma can better manage their symptoms and improve their quality of life. It is essential to maintain a clean and allergen-free living environment, monitor air quality, and take preventive measures during high-risk weather conditions. Additionally, regular medical check-ups and adherence to prescribed medications can help in effectively controlling asthma triggered by environmental factors.

Genetic Factors

Genetic factors play a crucial role in determining an individual's susceptibility to asthma. While asthma is not solely determined by genetics, family history and inherited traits can significantly increase the risk of developing the condition.

Here's an overview of genetic factors associated with asthma:

1. Family History: A strong family history of asthma or allergic conditions (such as hay fever and eczema) increases the likelihood of developing asthma. If one or both parents have asthma, a child is more likely to inherit genetic predispositions that contribute to asthma susceptibility.

2. Genetic Variants: Specific genetic variants and variations in genes related to immune responses and airway inflammation contribute to asthma susceptibility. **These include genes involved in:**

• Immune System Regulation: Genes that regulate the immune response, including those affecting the production of immunoglobulin E (IgE), cytokines, and other immune mediators.

• Airway Inflammation: Genes that influence inflammation in the airways, such as those affecting the production of inflammatory cytokines and chemokines.

• Airway Hyperresponsiveness: Genes that affect the responsiveness of airway smooth muscles and their contraction in response to stimuli.

3. Gene-Environment Interactions: Genetic factors interact with environmental exposures to influence asthma development and severity. Certain genetic variants may increase susceptibility to specific environmental triggers, such as allergens or air pollutants, leading to asthma symptoms.

Lifestyle Factors

While genetics plays a significant role in asthma susceptibility, lifestyle factors also contribute to the development and management of asthma. Adopting healthy lifestyle habits can help reduce the risk of asthma exacerbations and improve overall respiratory health.

Here are key lifestyle factors to consider:

1. Smoking and Secondhand Smoke: Smoking and exposure to secondhand smoke are significant risk factors for asthma. Smoking irritates the airways, increases inflammation, and reduces lung function, making asthma symptoms worse. Avoiding smoking and environments where smoking occurs is essential for asthma management.

2. Physical Activity and Exercise: Regular physical activity is beneficial for overall health, including respiratory health. However, for individuals with exercise-induced asthma (EIA), certain precautions may be necessary to prevent asthma symptoms during physical activity. These include warming up before exercise, using asthma medications as prescribed, and avoiding exercise in cold, dry air.

3. Diet and Nutrition: A healthy diet rich in fruits, vegetables, whole grains, and lean proteins can support immune function and reduce inflammation, which may help manage asthma symptoms. Some individuals with asthma may benefit from identifying and avoiding specific food triggers that worsen their symptoms.

4. Stress Management: Stress and strong emotions can trigger asthma symptoms in some individuals. Practicing stress management techniques such as deep breathing, meditation, yoga, and mindfulness can help reduce stress levels and improve asthma control.

5. Allergen Avoidance: Avoiding allergens that trigger asthma, such as pollen, dust mites, pet dander, and mold, is crucial for managing the condition. This includes using allergen-proof bedding, regularly cleaning indoor spaces, and minimizing exposure to pets if allergic.

6. Medication Adherence: Adhering to prescribed medications is essential for controlling asthma symptoms and preventing asthma attacks. This includes using daily long-term control medications as directed, carrying quick-relief inhalers for symptom relief, and following an asthma action plan provided by healthcare providers.

7. Environmental Control: Creating an asthma-friendly environment by maintaining good indoor air quality, reducing exposure to environmental pollutants (such as smoke and chemicals), and monitoring asthma triggers can help prevent asthma exacerbations.

By addressing genetic predispositions and adopting healthy lifestyle practices, individuals with asthma can effectively manage their condition and improve their quality of life. Consulting healthcare providers for personalized asthma management strategies and regular monitoring are essential components of comprehensive asthma care.

CHAPTER 6

The Role of Diet in Asthma Management

Diet plays a significant role in asthma management, influencing both the prevention of symptoms and the severity of asthma attacks. Understanding how diet affects asthma can empower individuals to make informed dietary choices that support respiratory health.

How Diet Affects Asthma

1. Inflammation Modulation:

• Certain foods can either promote or reduce inflammation in the body, including the airways. Chronic inflammation is a hallmark of asthma, contributing to airway narrowing and increased mucus production.

• Anti-inflammatory Foods: Foods rich in antioxidants, omega-3 fatty acids, and phytochemicals (such as fruits, vegetables, nuts, seeds, and fatty fish) have anti-inflammatory properties that may help reduce airway inflammation and improve asthma symptoms.

• Pro-inflammatory Foods: Conversely, a diet high in processed foods, trans fats, refined sugars, and excessive omega-6 fatty acids (found in vegetable oils) can promote inflammation and potentially worsen asthma symptoms.

2. Weight Management:

• Obesity is a risk factor for asthma and can exacerbate asthma symptoms due to increased inflammation, reduced lung function, and heightened responsiveness of the airways.

• A balanced diet that supports weight management, combined with regular physical activity, can help reduce the risk of developing asthma and improve asthma control in individuals who are overweight or obese.

3. Antioxidant Defense:

• Antioxidants protect cells from damage caused by free radicals, which are unstable molecules that contribute to inflammation and oxidative stress.

• Sources of Antioxidants: Foods rich in vitamins C and E, beta-carotene, selenium, and flavonoids (such as fruits, vegetables, nuts, seeds, and whole grains) support antioxidant defenses and may help mitigate oxidative stress in the airways.

4. Allergen Sensitivities:

• Some individuals with asthma also have food allergies or sensitivities that can trigger asthma symptoms.

• Common Allergenic Foods: Peanuts, tree nuts, shellfish, dairy products, and eggs are common allergens that may exacerbate asthma in sensitive individuals. Identifying and avoiding specific food triggers can help manage asthma symptoms.

5. Omega-3 and Omega-6 Balance:

• Omega-3 fatty acids (found in fatty fish like salmon, flaxseeds, and walnuts) have anti-inflammatory properties and may help reduce airway inflammation.

• Omega-6 fatty acids (found in vegetable oils, processed foods, and meats) can promote inflammation when consumed in excess. Balancing the intake of omega-3 and omega-6 fatty acids may support asthma management.

6. Dietary Fiber and Gut Health:

• Fiber-rich foods (such as fruits, vegetables, legumes, and whole grains) support gut health and may influence immune function and inflammation.

• A healthy gut microbiome is associated with reduced inflammation and improved respiratory health, potentially benefiting individuals with asthma.

7. Fluid Intake:

• Adequate hydration supports overall respiratory function by maintaining optimal mucous membrane hydration and reducing airway irritation.

• Water is the best choice for hydration, while sugary drinks and excessive caffeine intake should be limited, as they can potentially worsen asthma symptoms in some individuals.

Incorporating a balanced and nutritious diet plays a crucial role in managing asthma and promoting overall respiratory health. By focusing on anti-inflammatory foods, maintaining a healthy weight, managing allergen sensitivities, and supporting gut health, individuals with asthma can potentially reduce the frequency and severity of asthma symptoms. Consulting with healthcare providers and registered dietitians for personalized dietary recommendations is essential for optimizing asthma management strategies.

Overview of Diet and Respiratory Health

Diet plays a critical role in maintaining respiratory health, influencing both the prevention of respiratory conditions and the management of respiratory diseases such as asthma. Scientific studies provide valuable insights into how specific dietary patterns and nutrients impact respiratory function and overall lung health.

Scientific Studies and Evidence

1. Anti-inflammatory Diets:

• Mediterranean Diet: Research suggests that the Mediterranean diet, rich in fruits, vegetables, whole grains, nuts, seeds, and olive oil, is associated with reduced inflammation and improved lung function. Components such as omega-3 fatty acids, antioxidants (vitamins C and E, beta-carotene), and polyphenols may contribute to these benefits.

• DASH Diet (Dietary Approaches to Stop Hypertension): This diet emphasizes fruits, vegetables, low-fat dairy, whole grains, and lean proteins, and has shown potential benefits for reducing inflammation and improving lung health.

2. Omega-3 Fatty Acids:

• Omega-3 fatty acids, found in fatty fish (salmon, mackerel, sardines), flaxseeds, and walnuts, have anti-inflammatory properties. Studies suggest that omega-3 supplementation or increased dietary intake may help reduce airway inflammation and improve lung function in individuals with respiratory conditions.

3. Antioxidants:

• Vitamins C and E: These antioxidants protect lung tissue from oxidative stress caused by free radicals, potentially reducing inflammation and improving respiratory function.

• Beta-carotene: Found in orange and yellow fruits and vegetables (carrots, sweet potatoes, apricots), beta-carotene is converted into vitamin A in the body and supports lung health by enhancing immune function.

4. Vitamin D:

• Adequate vitamin D levels are associated with reduced risk of respiratory infections and improved lung function. Vitamin D may also modulate immune responses and reduce inflammation in the respiratory tract.

5. Probiotics and Gut Health:

• Emerging research suggests a link between gut health and respiratory health. Probiotics, beneficial bacteria found in fermented foods (yogurt, kefir, sauerkraut), may help regulate immune responses and reduce inflammation, potentially benefiting individuals with respiratory conditions.

6. Effects of Obesity and Weight Management:

• Obesity is a risk factor for respiratory conditions such as asthma and obstructive sleep apnea. Maintaining a healthy weight through a balanced diet and regular physical activity can reduce inflammation, improve lung function, and lower the risk of developing respiratory diseases.

7. Impact of Western Diet:

• The Western diet, characterized by high intake of processed foods, red meats, sugary beverages, and refined grains, is associated with increased inflammation and higher risk of respiratory diseases. Limiting these foods and emphasizing whole, unprocessed foods may help mitigate these risks.

Scientific evidence consistently supports the role of diet in maintaining respiratory health and managing respiratory conditions. Adopting a diet rich in anti-inflammatory foods, antioxidants, omega-3 fatty acids, and maintaining a healthy weight can contribute to improved lung function, reduced inflammation, and enhanced overall respiratory well-being. Individuals with respiratory conditions should consult healthcare providers or registered dietitians for personalized dietary recommendations tailored to their specific health needs and conditions.

CHAPTER 7

Foods That May Trigger Asthma

Certain foods can trigger asthma symptoms or exacerbate existing asthma in sensitive individuals. These triggers vary from person to person, and identifying and avoiding specific food allergens can help manage asthma more effectively.

Common Food Allergens

1. Peanuts and Tree Nuts:

• Peanuts and tree nuts (such as almonds, walnuts, cashews, and pistachios) are potent allergens that can trigger allergic reactions in some individuals. Symptoms may include wheezing, shortness of breath, and asthma exacerbations.

2. Shellfish:

• Shellfish, including shrimp, crab, lobster, and clams, are common allergens that can cause severe allergic reactions and potentially trigger asthma symptoms in sensitive individuals.

3. Dairy Products:

• Dairy products, such as milk, cheese, and yogurt, contain proteins (e.g., casein and whey) that some individuals may be allergic to. Dairy allergies can lead to respiratory symptoms, including asthma.

4. Eggs:

• Eggs are a common food allergen that can cause allergic reactions in both children and adults. Asthma symptoms may occur as part of an allergic reaction to eggs.

5. Wheat:

• Wheat allergies can trigger asthma symptoms in susceptible individuals. Wheat is present in many processed foods, baked goods, and cereals, making it essential for those with wheat allergies to read food labels carefully.

6. Soy:

• Soybeans and soy products are allergenic foods that can cause allergic reactions, including asthma symptoms, in sensitive individuals. Soy is commonly found in processed foods and soy-based products.

7. Fish:

• Certain types of fish, such as salmon, tuna, and cod, can trigger allergic reactions in some individuals. Asthma symptoms may occur as part of an allergic response to fish proteins.

Other Potential Triggers

In addition to common food allergens, some individuals may experience asthma symptoms or exacerbations in response to other foods or food additives.

These triggers can vary widely and may include:

• Sulfites: Preservatives found in dried fruits, wine, and processed foods can trigger asthma symptoms in sensitive individuals.

• Food Additives: Artificial colors, flavors, and preservatives added to processed foods may provoke asthma in some people.

• Cross-Reactivity: Some individuals with pollen allergies (e.g., to birch or ragweed pollen) may experience oral allergy syndrome, where certain raw fruits and vegetables trigger allergic reactions, including mild asthma symptoms.

Identifying and Managing Food Triggers

Managing asthma triggered by food allergens involves identifying specific triggers through allergy testing and keeping a food diary to track symptoms. Once identified, individuals should:

• Avoid Trigger Foods: Eliminate foods that trigger asthma symptoms from the diet.

• Read Labels Carefully: Check food labels for potential allergens and ingredients that may provoke asthma.

• Prepare Food Safely: Take precautions to avoid cross-contamination and accidental ingestion of allergenic foods.

• Consult Healthcare Providers: Seek guidance from allergists or healthcare providers to develop a personalized management plan and ensure adequate nutrition while avoiding trigger foods.

By identifying and managing food triggers effectively, individuals with asthma can reduce the frequency and severity of asthma symptoms, improve overall respiratory health, and enhance their quality of life.

Food Additives and Preservatives

Food additives and preservatives are substances added to food during processing or preparation to enhance flavor, appearance, texture, or shelf life. While generally considered safe, certain additives and preservatives may trigger asthma symptoms or exacerbate respiratory conditions in sensitive individuals.

Here are some case studies and examples highlighting their potential impact:

Sulfites

Case Study: Asthma Exacerbation from Sulfite Exposure

• Scenario: A 35-year-old woman with known asthma experiences severe wheezing and shortness of breath shortly after consuming dried fruits containing sulfites.

• Outcome: She presents to the emergency department and is treated with bronchodilators and corticosteroids to manage acute asthma exacerbation triggered by sulfite exposure.

Examples:

• Dried Fruits: Sulfites are commonly used in dried fruits to maintain color and prevent spoilage. Sensitive individuals, particularly those with asthma, may experience respiratory symptoms such as wheezing and coughing after consuming sulfite-containing dried fruits like apricots, raisins, and prunes.

• Wine: Sulfites are naturally present in wine and are also added as preservatives. Wine, especially white wine, can trigger asthma symptoms in individuals sensitive to sulfites.

Artificial Colors and Flavors

Case Study: Respiratory Symptoms Triggered by Food Coloring

• Scenario: A 10-year-old boy with asthma develops coughing and wheezing after consuming brightly colored candies containing artificial food dyes.

• Outcome: His symptoms worsen, requiring rescue inhaler use and a visit to his healthcare provider for asthma management.

Examples:

• Artificial Food Colors: Certain synthetic food dyes, such as tartrazine (Yellow 5) and Allura Red (Red 40), have been associated with allergic reactions and asthma exacerbations in sensitive individuals.

• Artificial Flavors: Some artificial flavors and flavor enhancers used in processed foods may contain compounds that trigger respiratory symptoms in susceptible individuals.

Monosodium Glutamate (MSG)

Case Study: Asthma Symptoms Linked to MSG Consumption

• Scenario: A 45-year-old man with a history of asthma experiences chest tightness and shortness of breath after consuming Chinese food containing monosodium glutamate (MSG) as a flavor enhancer.

• Outcome: He requires bronchodilator therapy to relieve acute respiratory distress attributed to MSG ingestion.

Examples:

• Processed Foods: MSG is commonly used in processed foods, soups, snacks, and Asian cuisine to enhance flavor. Some individuals with asthma may experience bronchoconstriction and respiratory discomfort after consuming foods containing MSG.

Nitrites and Nitrates

Case Study: Nitrite-Induced Respiratory Symptoms

• Scenario: A 50-year-old woman with asthma experiences exacerbation of respiratory symptoms after consuming processed meats preserved with nitrites and nitrates.

• Outcome: She requires increased use of rescue inhalers and visits her healthcare provider for asthma management.

Examples:

• Processed Meats: Nitrites and nitrates are commonly used in cured and processed meats (e.g., bacon, sausage, hot dogs) to prevent bacterial growth and maintain color. These compounds can potentially trigger asthma symptoms in sensitive individuals.

Managing Food Additives and Preservatives

For individuals with asthma or known sensitivities to food additives and preservatives, managing dietary intake involves:

• Reading Labels: Checking food labels for additives and preservatives that may trigger asthma symptoms.

• Avoidance: Limiting or avoiding foods known to contain triggers, such as sulfites in dried fruits and nitrites in processed meats.

• Personalized Approach: Consulting with healthcare providers or allergists to develop a personalized dietary plan that supports asthma management while ensuring adequate nutrition.

By understanding the potential impact of food additives and preservatives on respiratory health and taking proactive steps to manage dietary intake, individuals with asthma can minimize the risk of asthma exacerbations and maintain better control of their condition.

CHAPTER 8

Developing an Asthma-Friendly Diet

An asthma-friendly diet focuses on incorporating nutrients that support respiratory health, reduce inflammation, and potentially minimize asthma symptoms. Essential nutrients, including vitamins and minerals, play crucial roles in asthma management by enhancing lung function, supporting immune function, and reducing oxidative stress.

Essential Nutrients for Asthma Management

1. Vitamins

• Vitamin D: Adequate vitamin D levels are associated with reduced risk of asthma exacerbations and improved lung function. Sources include sunlight exposure and dietary sources like fatty fish (salmon, mackerel), egg yolks, and fortified foods (e.g., fortified milk, cereals).

• Vitamin C: Acts as an antioxidant that may help reduce inflammation and oxidative stress in the airways. Good sources include citrus fruits (oranges, grapefruits), strawberries, kiwi, bell peppers, and broccoli.

• Vitamin E: Another antioxidant that protects lung tissue from damage caused by free radicals. Sources include nuts (almonds, hazelnuts), seeds (sunflower seeds), spinach, and fortified cereals.

2. Minerals

• Magnesium: Helps relax the muscles around the bronchial tubes, potentially easing breathing. Good sources include leafy green vegetables (spinach, kale), nuts (almonds, cashews), seeds, and whole grains.

• Selenium: Acts as an antioxidant and may help reduce inflammation in the airways. Sources include Brazil nuts, seafood (oysters, tuna), lean meats, and whole grains.

• Zinc: Supports immune function and may help reduce respiratory infections that can trigger asthma exacerbations. Sources include lean meats (beef, poultry), seafood, beans, nuts, and whole grains.

Dietary Recommendations for Asthma-Friendly Nutrients

• Fruits and Vegetables: Aim for a variety of colorful fruits and vegetables daily to ensure intake of vitamins A, C, and E, as well as other beneficial phytochemicals and antioxidants.

• Omega-3 Fatty Acids: Found in fatty fish (salmon, mackerel, sardines), flaxseeds, and walnuts, omega-3s have anti-inflammatory properties that may help reduce airway inflammation.

• Lean Proteins: Choose lean sources of protein such as poultry, fish, beans, and legumes, which provide essential amino acids without the added saturated fats found in red meats.

• Whole Grains: Opt for whole grains like brown rice, quinoa, oats, and whole wheat, which provide fiber, B vitamins, and minerals like magnesium and selenium.

• Nuts and Seeds: Include a variety of nuts (almonds, walnuts) and seeds (flaxseeds, chia seeds) as sources of healthy fats, antioxidants, and minerals.

Practical Tips for Incorporating Asthma-Friendly Nutrients

• Smoothies: Blend fruits like berries and spinach with yogurt (if tolerated) or almond milk for a nutrient-packed breakfast or snack.

• Salads: Include a mix of colorful vegetables (bell peppers, tomatoes) and top with grilled chicken or chickpeas for added protein and fiber.

• Omega-3 Rich Meals: Enjoy baked or grilled salmon with a side of quinoa and steamed broccoli for a meal rich in omega-3s, magnesium, and vitamins.

• Snack Smart: Choose snacks like fresh fruit with a handful of nuts, or whole grain crackers with hummus, to boost nutrient intake throughout the day.

An asthma-friendly diet emphasizes nutrient-rich foods that support respiratory health, reduce inflammation, and provide essential vitamins and minerals. By incorporating a variety of fruits, vegetables, lean proteins, whole grains, and omega-3 rich foods, individuals with asthma can potentially improve lung function, manage symptoms more effectively, and enhance overall well-being. Consulting with a healthcare provider or registered dietitian can provide personalized guidance on optimizing nutrition for asthma management.

Antioxidants and Anti-inflammatory Compounds

Antioxidants and anti-inflammatory compounds play pivotal roles in asthma management by reducing oxidative stress, inflammation in the airways, and supporting overall respiratory health. Including foods rich in these compounds can potentially help mitigate asthma symptoms and improve lung function.

Antioxidants

1. Vitamin C:

• Acts as a powerful antioxidant that scavenges free radicals, reducing oxidative stress in the lungs and airways.

• Sources: Citrus fruits (oranges, lemons), strawberries, kiwi, bell peppers, broccoli, and tomatoes.

2. Vitamin E:

• Protects lung tissue from damage caused by oxidative stress and supports immune function.

• Sources: Nuts (almonds, hazelnuts), seeds (sunflower seeds), spinach, avocado, and fortified cereals.

3. Beta-carotene:

• Converted into vitamin A in the body, beta-carotene supports respiratory health and immune function.

• Sources: Carrots, sweet potatoes, spinach, kale, apricots, and mangoes.

4. Flavonoids:

• Plant compounds with antioxidant and anti-inflammatory properties that may help reduce airway inflammation.

• Sources: Berries (blueberries, strawberries), grapes, citrus fruits, apples, onions, and green tea.

Omega-3 Fatty Acids

Omega-3 fatty acids are essential fats known for their anti-inflammatory properties, which can help reduce inflammation in the airways and improve lung function in individuals with asthma.

1. Alpha-Linolenic Acid (ALA):

• Found in plant sources like flaxseeds, chia seeds, and walnuts.

• ALA can be converted in small amounts to EPA (eicosapentaenoic acid) and DHA (docosahexaenoic acid), which are more directly beneficial for reducing inflammation.

2. Eicosapentaenoic Acid (EPA) and Docosahexaenoic Acid (DHA):

• Found primarily in fatty fish such as salmon, mackerel, and sardines.

• EPA and DHA are directly associated with anti-inflammatory effects in the body, including the respiratory system.

Incorporating Antioxidants and Omega-3 Fatty Acids into Your Diet

• Salmon and Sardines: Enjoy grilled or baked fatty fish twice a week to boost intake of EPA and DHA.

• Flaxseeds and Chia Seeds: Add ground flaxseeds or chia seeds to smoothies, yogurt, or oatmeal for a plant-based source of ALA.

• Colorful Fruits and Vegetables: Include a variety of fruits and vegetables in your diet daily to benefit from a range of antioxidants like vitamin C, vitamin E, and beta-carotene.

• Nuts and Seeds: Snack on nuts (almonds, walnuts) and seeds (sunflower seeds) for a dose of vitamin E and ALA.

Practical Tips

• Smoothies: Blend spinach, berries, and a tablespoon of ground flaxseeds with yogurt or almond milk for a nutrient-packed antioxidant-rich breakfast.

• Salads: Create a colorful salad with mixed greens, bell peppers, tomatoes, and a drizzle of olive oil (rich in antioxidants) topped with grilled salmon or chicken.

• Snack Options: Opt for fresh fruit with a handful of nuts or seeds, or whole grain crackers with hummus, for a balanced snack rich in antioxidants and healthy fats.

Antioxidants and omega-3 fatty acids are essential components of an asthma-friendly diet, offering anti-inflammatory and protective benefits for respiratory health. By incorporating a variety of fruits, vegetables, fatty fish, nuts, seeds, and antioxidant-rich foods into your meals and snacks, you can potentially reduce inflammation in the airways, manage asthma symptoms more effectively, and support overall lung function. Consulting with a healthcare provider or registered dietitian can provide personalized recommendations to optimize your diet for asthma management.

CHAPTER 9

Foods to Include In Your Diet

Fruits and Vegetables

Fruits and vegetables are essential components of an asthma-friendly diet, providing a rich array of vitamins, minerals, antioxidants, and fiber that support respiratory health and overall well-being.

Here are some key fruits and vegetables to include:

Fruits

1. Citrus Fruits:

• Oranges: Rich in vitamin C, which helps reduce inflammation and supports immune function.

• Grapefruits, Lemons, and Limes: Also high in vitamin C and antioxidants that protect against oxidative stress.

2. Berries:

• Blueberries, Strawberries, Raspberries: Packed with antioxidants like vitamin C and flavonoids, which help combat inflammation and improve lung function.

3. Apples:

• Contain quercetin, a flavonoid with anti-inflammatory properties that may benefit lung health.

4. Bananas:

• Good source of vitamin B6, which may help reduce asthma symptoms by reducing inflammation.

5. Avocado:

• Provides vitamin E, potassium, and healthy monounsaturated fats that support lung health.

Vegetables

1. Leafy Greens:

• Spinach, Kale, Swiss Chard: Rich in magnesium, vitamin C, and antioxidants that help reduce inflammation and support lung function.

2. Bell Peppers:

• Excellent source of vitamin C and beta-carotene, which converts to vitamin A and supports respiratory health.

3. Broccoli and Brussels Sprouts:

• Cruciferous vegetables rich in antioxidants and fiber, which help reduce inflammation and support immune function.

4. Carrots and Sweet Potatoes:

• High in beta-carotene, which converts to vitamin A and supports lung health and immune function.

5. Tomatoes:

• Rich in vitamin C, lycopene, and antioxidants that help reduce inflammation and protect against oxidative stress.

Tips for Incorporating Fruits and Vegetables

• Smoothies: Blend spinach, kale, berries, and a banana with yogurt or almond milk for a nutrient-packed breakfast or snack.

• Salads: Create colorful salads with mixed greens, bell peppers, tomatoes, avocado, and a drizzle of olive oil (rich in antioxidants).

• Snacks: Enjoy fresh fruit with a handful of nuts or seeds, or raw vegetables with hummus, for a satisfying and nutritious snack.

Including a variety of fruits and vegetables in your daily diet provides essential nutrients, antioxidants, and fiber that support respiratory health and help manage asthma symptoms. Aim to eat a rainbow of colors to benefit from a wide range of vitamins, minerals, and phytochemicals that promote lung function and overall well-being. Consulting with a healthcare provider or registered dietitian can help tailor your diet to optimize asthma management and ensure you're meeting your nutritional needs effectively.

Lean Proteins

Lean proteins are essential for maintaining muscle health, supporting immune function, and providing sustained energy. Choosing lean sources of protein helps reduce intake of saturated fats, which can contribute to inflammation.

Here are some beneficial options:

1. Poultry:

• Chicken Breast: A lean source of protein that can be baked, grilled, or sautéed with herbs and spices for flavor.

• Turkey: Another lean option that provides protein and essential nutrients without excess fat.

2. Fish:

• Salmon, Trout, Mackerel: Fatty fish rich in omega-3 fatty acids, which have anti-inflammatory properties and support lung health.

• Cod, Tilapia: Lean white fish options that provide protein with lower fat content.

3. Legumes:

• Beans (Black beans, Kidney beans, Chickpeas): High in protein, fiber, and antioxidants. They can be included in soups, salads, or as a main dish.

• Lentils: Provide protein, fiber, and essential minerals like iron and folate. Great for soups, stews, and vegetarian dishes.

4. Tofu and Tempeh:

• Plant-based sources of protein that also provide calcium, iron, and magnesium. They can be stir-fried, grilled, or used in salads and wraps.

Whole Grains

Whole grains are rich in fiber, vitamins, minerals, and antioxidants, providing sustained energy and supporting overall health. Opt for whole grains over refined grains for maximum nutritional benefits:

1. Oats:

• High in soluble fiber, which helps stabilize blood sugar levels and promotes heart health. Can be enjoyed as oatmeal or added to smoothies.

2. Quinoa:

• Complete protein source containing all essential amino acids. It's versatile and can be used in salads, stir-fries, or as a side dish.

3. Brown Rice:

• Provides fiber, B vitamins, and minerals like magnesium and selenium. Ideal as a base for grain bowls, stir-fries, or alongside lean proteins.

4. Whole Wheat:

• Includes whole wheat bread, pasta, and couscous. These options provide fiber, B vitamins, and minerals that support digestive health and overall well-being.

Healthy Fats

Incorporating healthy fats into your diet is crucial for maintaining cell membranes, supporting brain health, and reducing inflammation. Opt for sources of unsaturated fats:

1. Nuts and Seeds:

• Almonds, Walnuts, Flaxseeds, Chia Seeds: Rich in omega-3 fatty acids, fiber, and antioxidants. They can be sprinkled on salads, yogurt, or eaten as a snack.

2. Avocado:

• Provides monounsaturated fats, fiber, potassium, and vitamin E. Enjoy sliced avocado on toast, in salads, or as a topping for soups.

3. Olive Oil:

• Contains monounsaturated fats and antioxidants. Use it for cooking, drizzling over salads, or as a dip for whole grain bread.

4. Fatty Fish:

• As mentioned earlier, salmon, trout, and mackerel are rich sources of omega-3 fatty acids that support heart health and reduce inflammation.

Tips for Incorporating Lean Proteins, Whole Grains, and Healthy Fats

• Meal Prep: Cook batches of lean proteins like chicken or beans, whole grains like quinoa or brown rice, and incorporate them into meals throughout the week.

• Balance Your Plate: Aim for a balanced plate with lean protein, whole grains, and plenty of vegetables to ensure a variety of nutrients in each meal.

• Healthy Snacks: Snack on a handful of nuts, Greek yogurt with berries, or whole grain crackers with avocado for a satisfying and nutritious snack.

Including lean proteins, whole grains, and healthy fats in your diet provides essential nutrients, promotes sustained energy, and supports overall health, including respiratory function. By choosing nutrient-dense foods and incorporating them into balanced meals and snacks, you can optimize your diet for asthma management and overall well-being. Consulting with a healthcare provider or registered dietitian can provide personalized guidance to help you achieve your nutritional goals and manage asthma effectively.

CHAPTER 10

Foods to Avoid

Processed Foods

Processed foods are generally high in unhealthy fats, refined sugars, and additives that can contribute to inflammation and worsen asthma symptoms. Avoiding these foods can help maintain better respiratory health and overall well-being.

Here are some types of processed foods to limit or avoid:

1. Fast Food:
• Burgers, fries, and other fast-food items are often high in trans fats, sodium, and refined carbohydrates, which can contribute to inflammation.

2. Packaged Snacks:

• Chips, crackers, cookies, and snack cakes are typically high in unhealthy fats, refined sugars, and artificial additives that can trigger inflammation and exacerbate asthma symptoms.

3. Processed Meats:

• Hot dogs, sausages, and deli meats often contain high levels of sodium, preservatives (like nitrates and nitrites), and unhealthy fats that can be detrimental to respiratory health.

4. Sugary Beverages:

• Sodas, energy drinks, and sugary fruit juices are high in refined sugars and can contribute to inflammation and weight gain, potentially worsening asthma symptoms.

5. Frozen Meals and Dinners:

• Convenience meals often contain high levels of sodium, unhealthy fats, and additives. These can contribute to inflammation and are generally low in essential nutrients.

Tips for Avoiding Processed Foods

• Read Labels: Check food labels for ingredients like hydrogenated oils, high-fructose corn syrup, and artificial additives. Choose foods with minimal processing and natural ingredients.

• Cook at Home: Prepare meals using fresh, whole ingredients whenever possible. This allows you to control the amount of unhealthy fats, sugars, and additives in your diet.

• Choose Whole Foods: Opt for whole fruits and vegetables, lean proteins, whole grains, and healthy fats instead of processed alternatives.

• Limit Dining Out: Reduce frequency of eating out at restaurants or fast-food establishments where processed foods are commonly served.

Limiting or avoiding processed foods can help reduce inflammation, manage asthma symptoms more effectively, and support overall health. By focusing on whole, nutrient-dense foods and minimizing intake of processed and refined foods, you can optimize your diet to promote respiratory health and well-being. Consulting with a healthcare provider or registered dietitian can provide personalized guidance on dietary choices that best support your asthma management plan.

Sugary Drinks and Snacks: Sugary drinks and snacks contribute to inflammation, weight gain, and can exacerbate asthma symptoms. Limiting or avoiding these items can support better respiratory health and overall well-being:

1. Sodas and Energy Drinks:

• High in refined sugars and often contain artificial additives, which can contribute to inflammation and worsen asthma symptoms.

2. Sweetened Fruit Juices:

• Even natural fruit juices can be high in sugars without the fiber content of whole fruits, leading to rapid spikes in blood sugar levels.

3. Sweetened Teas and Coffees:

• Flavored teas and coffee beverages with added sugars can increase inflammation and may trigger asthma symptoms in some individuals.

4. Candies and Sweets:

• Confectioneries like candies, chocolates, and sweet snacks are high in sugars and often lack nutritional value, contributing to inflammation and potential weight gain.

High-Sodium Foods: High-sodium foods can lead to fluid retention, increased blood pressure, and may worsen asthma symptoms. Avoiding excessive sodium intake can help manage asthma and overall health:

1. Processed Meats:

• Deli meats, sausages, and hot dogs are high in sodium and may contain preservatives that can trigger inflammation and respiratory issues.

2. Canned Soups and Ready-to-Eat Meals:

• Often high in sodium as a preservative. Opt for low-sodium varieties or prepare homemade soups with fresh ingredients.

3. Salty Snacks:

• Chips, pretzels, and salted nuts are high-sodium snacks that can contribute to fluid retention and inflammation, potentially exacerbating asthma symptoms.

4. Condiments and Sauces:

• Soy sauce, ketchup, barbecue sauce, and other condiments can be high in sodium. Choose low-sodium options or use them sparingly.

Tips for Reducing Sugary Drinks, Snacks, and High-Sodium Foods

• Drink Water: Opt for water as your primary beverage. Infuse it with fruits or herbs for added flavor without added sugars.

• Choose Fresh Fruits: Enjoy whole fruits instead of sugary snacks. They provide natural sweetness and fiber, which helps regulate blood sugar levels.

• Read Labels: Check nutrition labels for sodium content and choose low-sodium or sodium-free options whenever possible.

• Cook at Home: Prepare meals using fresh ingredients to control sodium intake and avoid hidden sugars found in processed foods.

Avoiding sugary drinks, snacks, and high-sodium foods can help manage inflammation, support asthma management, and promote overall health. By prioritizing whole, nutrient-dense foods and mindful consumption of fluids and snacks, you can optimize your diet to better support respiratory function and well-being. Consulting with a healthcare provider or registered dietitian can offer personalized guidance on dietary choices that align with your asthma management plan and overall health goals.

CHAPTER 11

Meal Planning and Recipes

Creating an Asthma-Friendly Meal Plan

Creating a meal plan that supports asthma management involves incorporating nutrient-dense foods, avoiding triggers, and ensuring balanced meals throughout the day. **Here's how to create an asthma-friendly meal plan:**

1. Focus on Fresh Ingredients: Choose whole, unprocessed foods such as fruits, vegetables, lean proteins, and whole grains. These foods are rich in vitamins, minerals, antioxidants, and fiber that support respiratory health.

2. Include Omega-3 Fatty Acids: Incorporate foods rich in omega-3 fatty acids, such as fatty fish (salmon, trout), flaxseeds, and walnuts. Omega-3s have anti-inflammatory properties that can help reduce asthma symptoms.

3. Limit Trigger Foods: Avoid processed foods, sugary snacks, high-sodium foods, and foods that may trigger allergies or sensitivities, such as dairy or gluten, if applicable.

4. Hydrate with Water: Drink plenty of water throughout the day to stay hydrated. Avoid sugary drinks and excessive caffeine, as they can contribute to dehydration and potentially worsen asthma symptoms.

5. Balanced Meals: Aim for balanced meals that include a source of lean protein, complex carbohydrates (whole grains), healthy fats, and plenty of vegetables or fruits. This balance helps stabilize blood sugar levels and supports overall health.

6. Plan Ahead: Plan your meals for the week in advance. This can help you make healthier choices and reduce the temptation to eat convenience or processed foods.

Tips for Meal Planning

• Batch Cooking: Prepare larger batches of meals and store portions in the refrigerator or freezer for easy reheating. This saves time during busy days and ensures you have nutritious meals readily available.

• Variety: Incorporate a variety of colors and textures into your meals. Different fruits and vegetables provide different nutrients and antioxidants that support respiratory health.

• Snack Smart: Choose healthy snacks such as fresh fruits, nuts, yogurt, or whole grain crackers with hummus. Avoid sugary snacks and opt for nutrient-dense options that provide sustained energy.

Here are some simple and nutritious recipes to include in your meal plan:

Breakfast: Greek Yogurt Parfait

Ingredients:

- Greek yogurt
- Fresh berries (blueberries, strawberries)
- Granola (low-sugar, whole grain)
- Honey (optional)

Instructions: Layer Greek yogurt with fresh berries and granola in a bowl or glass. Drizzle with honey if desired.

Lunch: Grilled Chicken Salad

Ingredients:

- Grilled chicken breast, sliced
- Mixed greens (spinach, kale)
- Cherry tomatoes, halved
- Cucumber, sliced
- Avocado, diced
- Olive oil and lemon juice dressing

Instructions: Toss mixed greens with cherry tomatoes, cucumber, and avocado. Top with grilled chicken slices and drizzle with olive oil and lemon juice dressing.

Dinner: Baked Salmon with Quinoa and Steamed Vegetables

Ingredients:

- Salmon filets
- Quinoa
- Broccoli and carrots, steamed
- Lemon wedges

Instructions: Season salmon with herbs and bake until cooked through. Serve with quinoa and steamed broccoli and carrots. Garnish with lemon wedges.

Creating an asthma-friendly meal plan involves choosing nutritious foods that support respiratory health, avoiding triggers, and maintaining balanced meals throughout the day. By planning ahead, incorporating a variety of nutrient-dense foods, and following these tips, you can optimize your diet to manage asthma effectively and promote overall well-being. Adjust your meal plan based on personal preferences and consult with a healthcare provider or registered dietitian for personalized guidance tailored to your specific needs and health goals.

Sample Weekly Meal Plans

Here are two sample weekly meal plans designed to support asthma management by focusing on nutrient-dense foods, avoiding triggers, and ensuring balanced meals throughout the day:

Meal Plan 1: Balanced and Nutritious
Monday:
• Breakfast: Greek Yogurt Parfait (Greek yogurt, fresh berries, granola)
• Lunch: Quinoa Salad with Grilled Chicken (quinoa, mixed greens, grilled chicken, cherry tomatoes, cucumber, olive oil and lemon dressing)
• Dinner: Baked Salmon with Steamed Broccoli and Brown Rice (salmon, broccoli, brown rice, lemon wedges)

Tuesday:

• Breakfast: Smoothie (spinach, banana, almond milk, chia seeds)

• Lunch: Whole Wheat Wrap with Turkey, Avocado, and Mixed Greens

• Dinner: Vegetarian Chili (kidney beans, tomatoes, bell peppers, onions, spices) served with Whole Grain Bread

Wednesday:

• Breakfast: Oatmeal with Fresh Berries and Almonds

• Lunch: Lentil Soup with Whole Grain Crackers

• Dinner: Stir-Fried Tofu with Quinoa and Steamed Vegetables (tofu, quinoa, mixed vegetables, soy sauce)

Thursday:

• Breakfast: Whole Grain Toast with Peanut Butter and Sliced Banana

• Lunch: Greek Salad with Chickpeas (mixed greens, cucumber, cherry tomatoes, olives, feta cheese, chickpeas, olive oil and lemon dressing)

• Dinner: Grilled Chicken with Sweet Potato and Asparagus

Friday:

• Breakfast: Scrambled Eggs with Spinach and Whole Grain Toast

• Lunch: Caprese Salad (tomatoes, fresh mozzarella, basil, olive oil, balsamic vinegar)

• Dinner: Baked Cod with Quinoa Pilaf and Steamed Green Beans (cod, quinoa, green beans, lemon wedges)

Saturday:

• Breakfast: Yogurt Bowl with Mixed Berries and Granola

• Lunch: Turkey and Avocado Sandwich on Whole Grain Bread with Side Salad

• Dinner: Vegetable Stir-Fry with Tofu and Brown Rice (tofu, mixed vegetables, soy sauce, brown rice)

Sunday:

• Breakfast: Whole Wheat Pancakes with Fresh Fruit Compote

• Lunch: Minestrone Soup with Whole Grain Bread

• Dinner: Grilled Salmon with Quinoa Salad (salmon, quinoa, mixed greens, cherry tomatoes, cucumber, olive oil and lemon dressing)

Grocery Shopping Guide

Here's a guide to help you shop for the ingredients needed for your asthma-friendly meals:

Proteins:
• Chicken breast
• Turkey breast
• Salmon filets
• Tofu
• Eggs

Grains:
• Quinoa
• Brown rice
• Whole grain bread
• Whole wheat wraps
• Whole grain crackers

Vegetables:

- Spinach

- Kale

- Broccoli

- Bell peppers

- Tomatoes

- Cucumber

- Asparagus

- Green beans

Fruits:

- Berries (blueberries, strawberries, raspberries)

- Bananas

- Avocado

- Lemons

Dairy and Alternatives:

- Greek yogurt

- Almond milk

Legumes:

- Chickpeas

• Lentils

• Kidney beans

Nuts and Seeds:

• Almonds

• Chia seeds

Other:

• Olive oil

• Balsamic vinegar

• Herbs and spices (oregano, basil, thyme, cumin)

• Fresh mozzarella (if desired for salads)

Tips for Grocery Shopping

• Plan Ahead: Make a list based on your meal plan to avoid impulse buys and ensure you have everything you need for healthy meals.

• Read Labels: Choose low-sodium options and avoid processed foods with added sugars and unhealthy fats.

• Shop the Perimeter: Focus on fresh produce, lean proteins, and whole grains found around the edges of the grocery store.

• Stock Up on Staples: Keep pantry essentials like whole grains, canned beans, and spices stocked for easy meal preparation.

By following these meal plans and shopping guide, you can support your asthma management goals with nutritious, balanced meals that promote overall health and well-being. Adjust recipes and ingredients based on personal preferences and consult with a healthcare provider or registered dietitian for personalized dietary advice tailored to your specific needs.

CHAPTER 12

Breakfast Recipes

Nutrient-Rich Smoothies

1. Green Power Smoothie

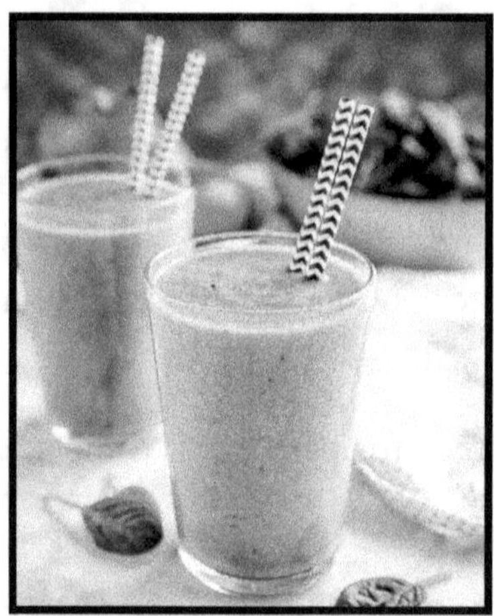

Ingredients:

- 1 cup spinach
- 1/2 cup kale
- 1 banana
- 1/2 cup Greek yogurt
- 1 tablespoon chia seeds

• 1/2 cup almond milk (unsweetened)

Instructions:

1. Blend spinach, kale, banana, Greek yogurt, chia seeds, and almond milk until smooth.

2. Add more almond milk if needed for desired consistency.

3. Pour into a glass and enjoy immediately.

2. Berry Blast Smoothie

Ingredients:

• 1 cup mixed berries (strawberries, blueberries, raspberries)

• 1/2 cup spinach

• 1/2 cup Greek yogurt

• 1 tablespoon flax seeds

• 1/2 cup coconut water

Instructions:

1. Combine mixed berries, spinach, Greek yogurt, flaxseeds, and coconut water in a blender.

2. Blend until smooth and creamy.

3. Serve chilled in a glass or bowl.

Anti-inflammatory Breakfast Bowls

1. Quinoa Breakfast Bowl

Ingredients:

- 1/2 cup cooked quinoa
- 1/2 cup mixed berries (blueberries, strawberries)
- 1/4 cup chopped nuts (almonds, walnuts)
- 1 tablespoon honey
- 1/2 cup Greek yogurt

Instructions:

1. In a bowl, layer cooked quinoa, mixed berries, and chopped nuts.

2. Drizzle with honey and top with Greek yogurt.

3. Serve immediately.

2. Turmeric Oatmeal Bowl

Ingredients:

- 1/2 cup rolled oats (cooked)
- 1/2 teaspoon ground turmeric
- 1/2 teaspoon cinnamon
- 1 tablespoon honey

- 1/2 cup almond milk (unsweetened)

- Fresh fruit (banana slices, berries)

Instructions:

1. Cook rolled oats with almond milk, turmeric, cinnamon, and honey until creamy.

2. Transfer to a bowl and top with fresh fruit.

3. Sprinkle with additional cinnamon if desired.

Whole Grain Options

1. Avocado Toast with Poached Egg

Ingredients:

- 1 slice whole grain bread (toasted)

- 1/2 avocado (mashed)

- 1 poached egg

- Salt and pepper to taste

Instructions:

1. Toast whole grain bread until golden brown.

2. Spread mashed avocado on top of the toast.

3. Top with a poached egg and season with salt and pepper.

2. Whole Grain Pancakes

Ingredients:

- 1 cup whole wheat flour
- 1 tablespoon baking powder
- 1/2 teaspoon salt
- 1 tablespoon honey or maple syrup
- 1 cup almond milk (unsweetened)
- 1 egg
- 1 tablespoon melted coconut oil

Instructions:

1. In a bowl, whisk together whole wheat flour, baking powder, and salt.

2. In another bowl, whisk honey or maple syrup, almond milk, egg, and melted coconut oil.

3. Combine wet and dry ingredients until smooth.

4. Heat a lightly oiled griddle or frying pan over medium-high heat.

5. Pour batter onto the griddle, using approximately 1/4 cup for each pancake.

6. Cook until bubbles form and edges are dry, then flip and cook until golden brown on the other side.

These breakfast recipes provide nutrient-rich options, anti-inflammatory ingredients, and whole grain choices to support your asthma management goals and promote overall health. Adjust recipes based on personal preferences and dietary needs, ensuring they align with your wellness plan. Enjoy these wholesome meals to start your day with energy and nutrition.

Lunch Recipes

Light and Healthy Salads

1. Mediterranean Chickpea Salad

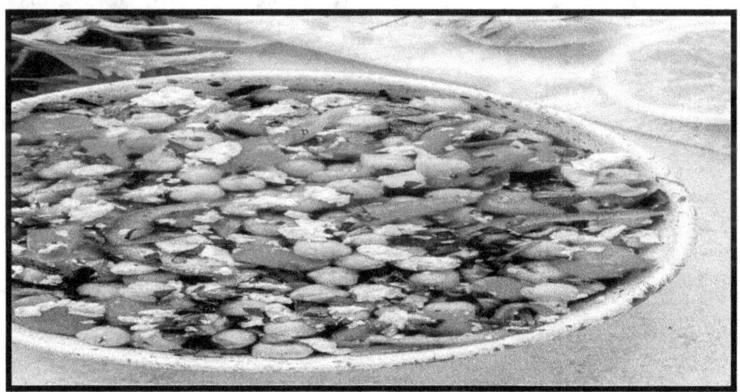

Ingredients:

- 1 can chickpeas (rinsed and drained)
- 1 cucumber (diced)
- 1 cup cherry tomatoes (halved)
- 1/4 cup red onion (thinly sliced)
- 1/4 cup Kalamata olives (pitted and sliced)
- 1/2 cup feta cheese (crumbled)
- 2 tablespoons fresh parsley (chopped)
- Juice of 1 lemon
- 2 tablespoons olive oil
- Salt and pepper to taste

Instructions:

1. In a large bowl, combine chickpeas, cucumber, cherry tomatoes, red onion, olives, feta cheese, and parsley.
2. Drizzle with lemon juice and olive oil.
3. Season with salt and pepper, toss gently to combine.
4. Serve chilled.

2. Asian Quinoa Salad

Ingredients:

- 1 cup cooked quinoa

- 1 cup shredded red cabbage

- 1 carrot (shredded)

- 1/2 cup edamame (cooked)

- 1/4 cup cilantro (chopped)

- 1/4 cup peanuts (chopped)

- 2 tablespoons sesame seeds

- 2 tablespoons soy sauce

- 1 tablespoon rice vinegar

- 1 tablespoon honey

- 1 teaspoon sesame oil

Instructions:

1. In a large bowl, combine cooked quinoa, red cabbage, carrot, edamame, cilantro, peanuts, and sesame seeds.

2. In a small bowl, whisk together soy sauce, rice vinegar, honey, and sesame oil.

3. Pour dressing over salad and toss gently to combine.

4. Serve chilled or at room temperature.

Protein-Packed Wraps and Sandwiches

1. Turkey and Avocado Wrap

Ingredients:

- Whole wheat wrap
- 4 slices turkey breast
- 1/2 avocado (sliced)
- Handful of mixed greens

Instructions:

1. Lay the whole wheat wrap flat.

2. Layer turkey breast slices, avocado slices, and mixed greens in the center of the wrap.

3. Fold in the sides of the wrap and roll tightly.

4. Cut in half and serve.

2. Caprese Sandwich

Ingredients:

- Whole grain bread
- Fresh mozzarella cheese (sliced)
- Tomato (sliced)
- Fresh basil leaves
- Balsamic glaze

Instructions:

1. Toast whole grain bread slices until golden brown.

2. Layer fresh mozzarella slices, tomato slices, and basil leaves on one slice of bread.

3. Drizzle with balsamic glaze.

4. Top with the second slice of bread and cut in half to serve.

Asthma-Friendly Soups

1. Lentil and Vegetable Soup

Ingredients:

- 1 cup lentils (rinsed)
- 1 onion (chopped)
- 2 carrots (diced)
- 2 celery stalks (diced)
- 1 zucchini (diced)
- 4 cups vegetable broth
- 1 teaspoon dried thyme
- Salt and pepper to taste

Instructions:

1. In a large pot, sauté onion, carrots, and celery until softened.

2. Add lentils, zucchini, vegetable broth, and dried thyme.

3. Bring to a boil, then reduce heat and simmer until lentils are tender, about 20-25 minutes.

4. Season with salt and pepper to taste.

5. Serve hot.

2. Chicken and Vegetable Noodle Soup

Ingredients:

- 1 tablespoon olive oil
- 1 onion (chopped)
- 2 carrots (sliced)
- 2 celery stalks (sliced)
- 1 garlic clove (minced)
- 6 cups chicken broth
- 2 cups cooked chicken (shredded)
- 1 cup egg noodles
- 1 teaspoon dried thyme
- Salt and pepper to taste

Instructions:

1. In a large pot, heat olive oil over medium heat.

2. Sauté onion, carrots, celery, and garlic until softened.

3. Add chicken broth, shredded chicken, egg noodles, and dried thyme.

4. Bring to a boil, then reduce heat and simmer until noodles are tender, about 10-12 minutes.

5. Season with salt and pepper to taste.

6. Serve hot.

These lunch recipes provide a variety of options that are light, protein-packed, and asthma-friendly, incorporating nutrient-dense ingredients and minimizing potential triggers. Enjoy these delicious meals to support your health and well-being throughout the day.

Dinner Recipes

Balanced and Nutritious Entrees

1. Grilled Salmon with Quinoa Pilaf

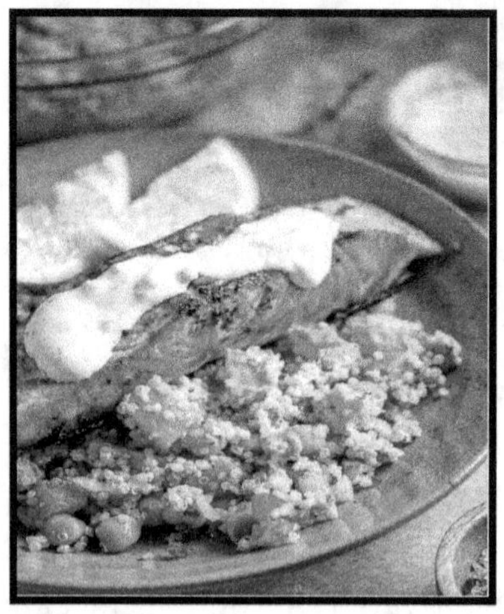

Ingredients:

- 4 salmon filets
- 1 cup quinoa
- 2 cups vegetable broth
- 1 tablespoon olive oil
- 1 lemon (juiced)
- Salt and pepper to taste

Instructions:

1. Rinse quinoa under cold water.

2. In a saucepan, bring vegetable broth to a boil.

3. Add quinoa, reduce heat to low, cover, and simmer for 15-20 minutes or until liquid is absorbed.

4. Meanwhile, preheat the grill to medium-high heat.

5. Brush salmon filets with olive oil, lemon juice, salt, and pepper.

6. Grill salmon for 4-5 minutes per side or until cooked through.

7. Serve grilled salmon over quinoa pilaf.

2. Turkey Meatballs with Whole Wheat Pasta

Ingredients:

- 1 lb ground turkey
- 1/2 cup breadcrumbs
- 1 egg
- 1/4 cup grated Parmesan cheese
- 1 teaspoon dried oregano
- 1 teaspoon garlic powder
- Salt and pepper to taste
- 1 jar marinara sauce
- 8 oz whole wheat pasta

Instructions:

1. Preheat the oven to 400°F (200°C).

2. In a bowl, combine ground turkey, breadcrumbs, egg, Parmesan cheese, oregano, garlic powder, salt, and pepper.

3. Shape mixture into meatballs and place on a baking sheet lined with parchment paper.

4. Bake meatballs for 20-25 minutes or until cooked through.

5. Meanwhile, cook whole wheat pasta according to package instructions.

6. Heat marinara sauce in a large skillet.

7. Add cooked meatballs to the skillet with marinara sauce and simmer for 5 minutes.

8. Serve meatballs and sauce over whole wheat pasta.

Vegetable-Forward Dishes

1. Ratatouille

Ingredients:

- 1 eggplant (cubed)
- 2 zucchinis (sliced)
- 1 yellow bell pepper (sliced)
- 1 red bell pepper (sliced)
- 1 onion (sliced)

- 4 garlic cloves (minced)
- 2 cups tomato sauce
- 1 tablespoon olive oil
- 1 teaspoon dried thyme
- Salt and pepper to taste

Instructions:

1. Preheat the oven to 375°F (190°C).

2. In a large baking dish, combine eggplant, zucchinis, bell peppers, onion, garlic, olive oil, dried thyme, salt, and pepper.

3. Roast vegetables in the oven for 30-40 minutes or until tender.

4. Remove from the oven and stir in tomato sauce.

5. Serve hot as a side dish or over cooked quinoa or brown rice.

2. Stir-Fried Tofu with Vegetables

Ingredients:

- 1 block tofu (firm or extra firm, cubed)
- 2 cups mixed vegetables (broccoli, bell peppers, snap peas)

- 2 tablespoons soy sauce
- 1 tablespoon hoisin sauce
- 1 tablespoon sesame oil
- 2 garlic cloves (minced)
- 1 tablespoon grated ginger
- Cooked brown rice

Instructions:

1. Heat sesame oil in a large skillet or wok over medium-high heat.

2. Add tofu cubes and stir-fry until golden brown on all sides, about 5-7 minutes.

3. Add mixed vegetables, garlic, and ginger to the skillet.

4. Stir-fry for another 3-4 minutes until vegetables are tender-crisp.

5. Stir in soy sauce and hoisin sauce, tossing to combine.

6. Serve stir-fried tofu and vegetables over cooked brown rice.

Omega-3 Rich Meals

1. Baked Cod with Lemon and Herbs

Ingredients:

- 4 cod filets

- 1 lemon (sliced)

- 2 tablespoons olive oil

- 2 garlic cloves (minced)

- 1 teaspoon dried dill

- Salt and pepper to taste

Instructions:

1. Preheat the oven to 400°F (200°C).

2. Place cod filets in a baking dish lined with parchment paper.

3. Drizzle olive oil over cod filets.

4. Sprinkle minced garlic, dried dill, salt, and pepper evenly over cod filets.

5. Arrange lemon slices on top of each cod filet.

6. Bake cod in the preheated oven for 15-20 minutes or until fish flakes easily with a fork.

7. Serve baked cod with steamed vegetables or a side salad.

2. Walnut-Crusted Salmon

Ingredients:

- 4 salmon filets
- 1/2 cup walnuts (chopped)
- 1/4 cup breadcrumbs
- 1 tablespoon Dijon mustard
- 1 tablespoon maple syrup
- 1 tablespoon olive oil

Instructions:

1. Preheat the oven to 375°F (190°C).

2. In a bowl, combine chopped walnuts, breadcrumbs, Dijon mustard, maple syrup, and olive oil.

3. Place salmon filets on a baking sheet lined with parchment paper.

4. Press walnut mixture onto the top of each salmon filet.

5. Bake salmon in the preheated oven for 12-15 minutes or until the fish flakes easily with a fork.

6. Serve walnut-crusted salmon with roasted vegetables or quinoa.

These dinner recipes offer balanced and nutritious options, vegetable-forward dishes, and meals rich in omega-3 fatty acids to support your asthma-friendly diet.

Enjoy these flavorful and wholesome meals as part of your evening routine, ensuring they align with your dietary preferences and wellness goals.

Snack and Dessert Recipes

Healthy Snack Ideas

1. Greek Yogurt with Berries

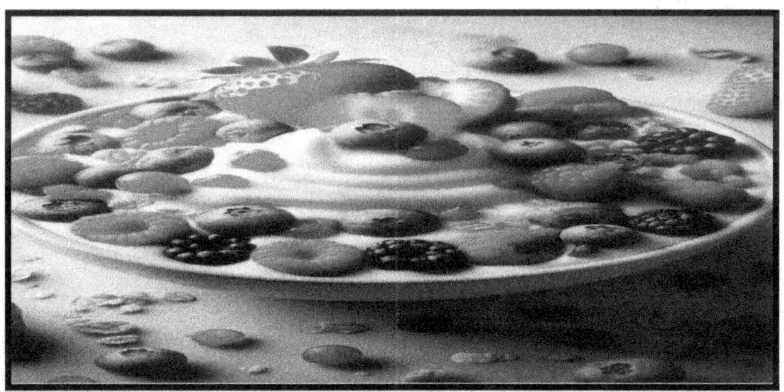

Ingredients:

• 1 cup plain Greek yogurt

• 1/2 cup mixed berries (strawberries, blueberries, raspberries)

• 1 tablespoon honey (optional)

Instructions:

1. In a bowl, spoon Greek yogurt.

2. Top with mixed berries.

3. Drizzle with honey if desired.

4. Enjoy as a refreshing and protein-packed snack.

2. Hummus and Veggie Sticks

Ingredients:

- 1/2 cup hummus

- Carrot sticks, cucumber slices, bell pepper strips

Instructions:

1. Arrange hummus in a small bowl.

2. Serve with carrot sticks, cucumber slices, and bell pepper strips.

3. Dip and enjoy this crunchy and nutritious snack.

Low-Sugar Desserts

1. Baked Apple Slices

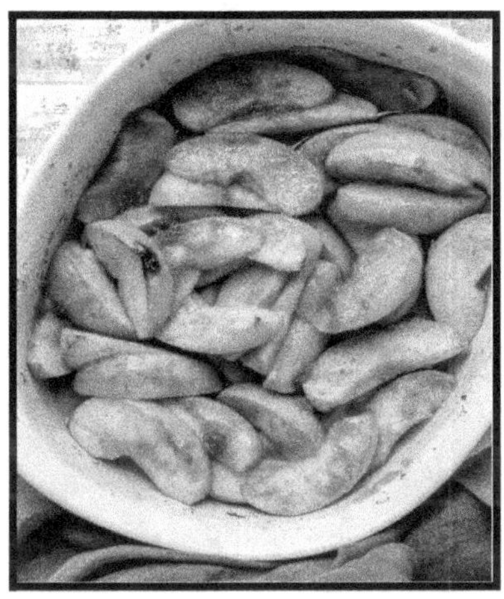

Ingredients:

- 2 apples (cored and sliced)
- 1 teaspoon cinnamon
- 1 tablespoon honey (optional)

Instructions:

1. Preheat the oven to 350°F (175°C).

2. Arrange apple slices on a baking sheet lined with parchment paper.

3. Sprinkle cinnamon over apple slices.

4. Drizzle with honey if desired.

5. Bake for 15-20 minutes or until the apples are tender.

6. Serve warm as a comforting low-sugar dessert.

2. Chia Seed Pudding

Ingredients:

• 1/4 cup chia seeds

• 1 cup unsweetened almond milk (or any milk of choice)

• 1 tablespoon maple syrup (optional)

• Fresh fruit for topping (e.g., berries, mango)

Instructions:

1. In a bowl, combine chia seeds and almond milk.

2. Stir well and let sit for 5 minutes.

3. Stir again to break up any clumps of chia seeds.

4. Cover and refrigerate for at least 2 hours or overnight until thickened.

5. Sweeten with maple syrup if desired.

6. Serve chilled, topped with fresh fruit.

Anti-inflammatory Snacks

1. Turmeric Roasted Chickpeas

Ingredients:

• 1 can chickpeas (rinsed and drained)

- 1 tablespoon olive oil

- 1 teaspoon ground turmeric

- 1/2 teaspoon ground cumin

- 1/2 teaspoon paprika

- Salt to taste

Instructions:

1. Preheat the oven to 400°F (200°C).

2. Pat chickpeas dry with a paper towel.

3. In a bowl, toss chickpeas with olive oil, turmeric, cumin, paprika, and salt.

4. Spread chickpeas in a single layer on a baking sheet lined with parchment paper.

5. Roast for 20-25 minutes, shaking the pan halfway through, until chickpeas are crispy.

6. Let cool slightly before serving as a crunchy and anti-inflammatory snack.

2. Avocado Toast with Turmeric

Ingredients:

- 1 ripe avocado

- 2 slices whole grain bread (toasted)

- 1/2 teaspoon ground turmeric
- Pinch of salt

Instructions:

1. Mash avocado in a bowl until smooth.

2. Stir in ground turmeric and salt.

3. Spread avocado mixture evenly onto toasted whole grain bread slices.

4. Serve immediately as a satisfying and anti-inflammatory snack.

These snack and dessert recipes offer a variety of options that are healthy, low in sugar, and incorporate anti-inflammatory ingredients to support your asthma-friendly diet. Enjoy these flavorful and nutritious treats throughout the day, ensuring they align with your dietary preferences and wellness goals.

CHAPTER 13

CHAPTER 13

Lifestyle and Asthma Management

Exercise and Physical Activity

Regular exercise and physical activity play crucial roles in managing asthma by improving lung function, overall fitness, and reducing asthma symptoms.

Here's a comprehensive look at integrating exercise into your asthma management plan:

Understanding Exercise-Induced Asthma (EIA):

• Definition: Exercise-induced asthma (EIA) refers to the narrowing of the airways during or after physical exertion, causing asthma symptoms like coughing, wheezing, or shortness of breath.

• Triggers: Cold, dry air or allergens encountered during exercise can trigger EIA.

• Management: Warm-up properly before exercise, use prescribed medications, and choose activities less likely to trigger symptoms (e.g., swimming or walking).

Types of Asthma-Friendly Exercises:

• Aerobic Exercises: Activities like walking, cycling (especially indoors), and swimming are generally well-tolerated.

• Yoga and Tai Chi: These practices emphasize controlled breathing and relaxation, which can benefit asthma management.

• Strength Training: Light to moderate resistance training can improve overall fitness without triggering asthma symptoms.

Tips for Exercising Safely with Asthma:

• Consult Your Doctor: Before starting any exercise program, consult your healthcare provider to tailor recommendations to your specific asthma condition.

• Warm-Up and Cool Down: Gradually warm up and cool down to prepare and recover your muscles and respiratory system.

• Monitor Symptoms: Be aware of early signs of asthma symptoms during exercise and adjust intensity or activity as needed.

• Stay Hydrated: Drink water before, during, and after exercise to maintain hydration, which supports respiratory function.

Incorporating Exercise into Daily Life:

• Consistency: Aim for at least 150 minutes of moderate-intensity aerobic activity per week, spread across several days.

• Variety: Mix different types of exercises to maintain interest and target different muscle groups.

• Environmental Considerations: Avoid exercising outdoors in cold or polluted environments that may exacerbate asthma symptoms.

By incorporating regular exercise and physical activity into your daily routine, you can effectively manage asthma symptoms, improve overall fitness, and enhance your quality of life. Always prioritize safety and consult your healthcare provider for personalized exercise recommendations tailored to your asthma management plan.

Benefits of Exercise for Asthma

Regular exercise offers numerous benefits for individuals managing asthma, contributing to overall health and well-being while specifically addressing asthma-related concerns. Here's an in-depth look at how exercise can positively impact asthma management:

1. Improved Lung Function:
• Mechanisms: Exercise strengthens respiratory muscles, increases lung capacity, and enhances overall breathing efficiency.
• Benefits: Improved lung function leads to better oxygen delivery, reduced breathlessness, and enhanced tolerance to physical exertion.

2. Enhanced Asthma Control:

• Reduced Symptoms: Regular physical activity can decrease the frequency and severity of asthma symptoms such as wheezing, coughing, and shortness of breath.

• Better Management: Exercise promotes better asthma control by minimizing airway inflammation and improving bronchodilation.

3. Weight Management:

• Healthy Body Weight: Maintaining a healthy weight through exercise reduces asthma severity and lowers the risk of obesity-related asthma complications.

• Support for Airways: Reduced weight decreases the strain on the respiratory system, facilitating easier breathing.

4. Reduced Inflammation:

• Anti-inflammatory Effects: Physical activity triggers anti-inflammatory responses in the body, potentially reducing airway inflammation associated with asthma.

• Improved Immunity: Enhanced immune function from regular exercise may lessen susceptibility to respiratory infections that can exacerbate asthma.

5. Psychological Benefits:

• Stress Reduction: Exercise helps manage stress and anxiety, which can trigger or worsen asthma symptoms.

• Enhanced Mental Health: Improved mood and mental well-being contribute to overall asthma management and quality of life.

Recommended Activities and Precautions

When integrating exercise into your asthma management plan, consider these recommended activities and precautions to ensure safe and effective participation:

1. Recommended Activities:

• Aerobic Exercises: Walking, cycling (especially stationary bikes), swimming, and water aerobics are generally well-tolerated.

• Yoga and Tai Chi: These practices emphasize controlled breathing and relaxation techniques beneficial for asthma management.

• Moderate Intensity: Engage in activities that elevate your heart rate without triggering asthma symptoms excessively.

2. Precautions:

• Warm-Up and Cool Down: Always warm up and cool down to prepare and recover your muscles and respiratory system.

• Stay Hydrated: Drink water before, during, and after exercise to maintain hydration, supporting optimal respiratory function.

• Know Your Limits: Be aware of your asthma triggers and symptoms. Modify activities or intensity if you experience any signs of asthma exacerbation.

• Weather Considerations: Exercise indoors during cold weather to avoid exposure to cold, dry air which can trigger asthma symptoms.

3. Consult Your Healthcare Provider:

• Individualized Plan: Discuss with your doctor or asthma specialist to develop an exercise plan tailored to your asthma severity and overall health.

• Medication Use: Ensure you have quick-relief medication (e.g., inhalers) readily available during exercise, as prescribed by your healthcare provider.

By incorporating recommended activities and observing necessary precautions, you can harness the benefits of exercise to effectively manage asthma, improve lung function, and enhance overall well-being. Always prioritize safety and consult your healthcare provider for personalized guidance on integrating exercise into your asthma management regimen.

CHAPTER 14

Stress Management

Stress can significantly impact asthma, exacerbating symptoms and triggering episodes. Managing stress effectively is crucial for asthma management and overall well-being.

Here's a comprehensive guide to understanding stress and its management in relation to asthma:

The Impact of Stress on Asthma

1. Asthma Triggers:

• Airway Sensitivity: Stress can lead to airway inflammation and increased sensitivity, making asthma symptoms more likely to occur.

• Breathing Patterns: Stress may cause shallow breathing or hyperventilation, which can trigger or worsen asthma attacks.

• Immune Response: Chronic stress weakens the immune system, making individuals more susceptible to respiratory infections that can exacerbate asthma.

2. Psychological Impact:

• Anxiety and Fear: Living with asthma can lead to anxiety about potential attacks, which can, in turn, increase stress levels and worsen symptoms.

• Quality of Life: Chronic stress related to asthma can affect daily activities, sleep patterns, and overall quality of life.

Techniques for Reducing Stress: Effective stress management techniques can help alleviate asthma symptoms and improve overall well-being. Incorporate these strategies into your daily routine:

1. Mindfulness and Relaxation Techniques:

• Deep Breathing: Practice diaphragmatic breathing or deep breathing exercises to promote relaxation and reduce stress-induced hyperventilation.

• Meditation and Mindfulness: Engage in mindfulness practices such as meditation or progressive muscle relaxation to calm the mind and reduce anxiety.

2. Physical Activity:

• Exercise: Regular physical activity not only improves lung function but also releases endorphins that help reduce stress and anxiety.

• Yoga and Tai Chi: These practices combine physical movement with relaxation techniques, fostering a sense of calm and reducing stress levels.

3. Cognitive Behavioral Therapy (CBT):

• Stress Management Techniques: CBT techniques, such as cognitive restructuring and stress inoculation training, can help individuals manage stressors related to asthma.

• Problem-Solving Skills: Learn effective problem-solving skills to tackle stressors and reduce their impact on asthma management.

4. Social Support:

• Support Network: Seek support from friends, family, or support groups to share experiences and receive emotional support.

• Open Communication: Discuss concerns and feelings with loved ones or a therapist to alleviate stress and promote a sense of control over asthma management.

5. Healthy Lifestyle Habits:

• Sleep Hygiene: Prioritize adequate sleep to reduce stress levels and support overall health.

• Nutrition: Maintain a balanced diet rich in fruits, vegetables, and whole grains to support immune function and overall well-being.

6. Relaxation Techniques:

• Progressive Muscle Relaxation: Tense and relax muscle groups sequentially to release physical tension and promote relaxation.

• Visualization: Use guided imagery or visualization techniques to create calming mental images and reduce stress responses.

Incorporating Stress Management into Daily Life

• Routine: Establish a daily routine that includes stress-reducing activities such as mindfulness exercises, physical activity, and relaxation techniques.

• Self-Care: Prioritize self-care activities that promote relaxation and emotional well-being, such as hobbies, reading, or spending time in nature.

• Flexibility: Be flexible and adaptable in managing stress, adjusting techniques based on individual needs and stressors.

By implementing these stress management techniques consistently, individuals with asthma can reduce the impact of stress on their condition, improve asthma control, and enhance overall quality of life. Regularly assess and adjust your stress management strategies to find what works best for you in managing asthma-related stress effectively.

Environmental Factors

Environmental factors play a significant role in asthma management, influencing both indoor and outdoor air quality. Creating an asthma-friendly environment at home and managing outdoor triggers are crucial steps in reducing asthma symptoms and improving overall respiratory health.

Creating an Asthma-Friendly Home

1. Indoor Air Quality:

• Allergen Control: Reduce exposure to common allergens such as dust mites, pet dander, mold, and pollen.

• Use allergen-proof mattress and pillow covers.

• Wash bedding regularly in hot water.

• Vacuum carpets and upholstery frequently use a vacuum cleaner with a HEPA filter.

• Keep indoor humidity levels below 50% to prevent mold growth.

• Air Filtration: Use high-efficiency air filters in HVAC systems and portable air purifiers to trap airborne allergens and pollutants.

• Ventilation: Ensure adequate ventilation in bathrooms, kitchens, and living areas to reduce indoor air pollutants and maintain fresh air circulation.

2. Reducing Irritants and Chemicals:

• Avoid Smoking: Prohibit smoking indoors and near windows to prevent exposure to secondhand smoke, a potent asthma trigger.

• Limit Harsh Chemicals: Use non-toxic cleaning products, paints, and household chemicals to minimize respiratory irritation.

• Natural Ventilation: Open windows when weather permits to improve indoor air exchange and reduce concentrations of indoor pollutants.

3. Bedroom Environment:

• Optimal Sleeping Conditions: Create a clean and allergen-free sleeping environment.

• Use hypoallergenic pillows and bedding.

• Remove stuffed animals and clutter from the bedroom.

• Keep windows closed during high pollen seasons or use pollen-proof window filters.

Managing Outdoor Triggers

1. Pollen and Outdoor Allergens:

• Monitor Pollen Counts: Check local pollen forecasts and limit outdoor activities during peak pollen times.

• Outdoor Clothing: Change clothes and shower after spending time outdoors during high pollen seasons to reduce allergen exposure.

• Landscaping: Choose low-allergen plants for landscaping and gardening to minimize pollen exposure around the home.

2. Air Pollution:

• Avoid Busy Roads: Limit outdoor exercise and activities near high-traffic areas where air pollution levels are elevated.

• Check Air Quality Index (AQI): Monitor AQI levels and plan outdoor activities accordingly to minimize exposure to pollutants.

3. Indoor-Outdoor Transition:

• Entryway Control: Place doormats at entryways and encourage family members to remove shoes to prevent tracking outdoor pollutants indoors.

• Pets and Allergens: Bathe pets regularly and keep them off furniture and out of bedrooms to reduce indoor allergen exposure.

By implementing these strategies to create an asthma-friendly home and manage outdoor triggers, individuals with asthma can significantly reduce exposure to allergens and irritants that exacerbate symptoms. Consistently maintaining good indoor air quality and minimizing outdoor triggers supports asthma management efforts, improves respiratory health, and enhances overall quality of life. Regularly assess and update environmental controls to ensure ongoing asthma symptom control and respiratory well-being.

CHAPTER 15

Personal Stories and Expert Advice

Real-life Stories

Sharing personal stories from individuals who have successfully managed asthma can provide inspiration, practical insights, and encouragement for others facing similar challenges.

Here are some real-life stories that highlight experiences, strategies, and lessons learned in managing asthma:

1. Emma's Journey to Asthma Control:

• Background: Emma, a 32-year-old graphic designer, shares her journey with asthma since childhood.

• Challenges: Emma struggled with frequent asthma attacks during her teens and early adulthood, impacting her daily life and career.

• Turning Point: After consulting with her healthcare provider, Emma developed a personalized asthma management plan that included daily controller medications, regular check-ups, and identifying triggers.

• Success: By diligently following her treatment plan and making lifestyle adjustments, such as avoiding smoke-filled environments and practicing stress management techniques, Emma achieved better asthma control. She now enjoys an active lifestyle and pursues her career without the fear of asthma attacks.

2. David's Experience with Exercise-induced Asthma (EIA):

• Background: David, a 45-year-old fitness enthusiast and marathon runner, discusses managing exercise-induced asthma.

• Diagnosis: David discovered he had EIA after experiencing wheezing and shortness of breath during intense workouts.

• Management Strategies: With guidance from his doctor, David incorporates a thorough warm-up routine, uses his rescue inhaler before exercise, and chooses low-allergen environments for outdoor runs.

• Achievements: Despite his initial setbacks, David successfully completed multiple marathons by adapting his training regimen and listening to his body's signals.

Expert Advice

Expert advice from healthcare professionals, asthma specialists, and researchers provides valuable guidance on asthma management strategies, treatment options, and lifestyle adjustments.

Here are insights from experts in the field:

1. Dr. Sarah Lopez, Allergist and Immunologist:

• Key Recommendations: "For individuals with asthma, it's crucial to work closely with your healthcare provider to develop a personalized asthma action plan. This plan should include daily medications, trigger identification and avoidance strategies, and emergency response guidelines."

• Empowerment through Education: "Education plays a pivotal role in asthma management. Understanding your asthma triggers, knowing how to use inhalers correctly, and recognizing early warning signs of an asthma exacerbation empowers individuals to take proactive steps in controlling their condition."

2. Prof. Michael Brown, Pulmonologist:

• On Lifestyle Adjustments: "In addition to medications, lifestyle modifications such as maintaining a healthy weight, avoiding smoke exposure, and managing stress effectively can significantly impact asthma control."

• Integration of Technology: "Advances in digital health tools, like asthma management apps and peak flow meters, allow individuals to monitor their asthma symptoms more closely and communicate effectively with their healthcare team.

Personal stories from individuals like Emma and David illustrate the diverse experiences of living with asthma and navigating its challenges. Expert advice emphasizes the importance of personalized care, education, and proactive management strategies. By sharing personal stories and expert insights, we aim to inspire others with asthma to take control of their health, seek support, and implement effective strategies for managing their condition successfully.

Interviews with Asthma Patients

1. Interview with Emily Parker:

Background:

• Emily Parker, a 28-year-old teacher, was diagnosed with asthma at the age of 10.

• Despite facing numerous challenges, she has managed to maintain a fulfilling and active lifestyle.

Interview Excerpts:

• Q: How did you first learn you had asthma?

• Emily: "I was always getting short of breath during PE classes. After several visits to the doctor, I was diagnosed with asthma. It was scary at first, but understanding what was happening to me made a big difference."

• Q: What strategies have helped you manage your asthma effectively?

• Emily: "Staying active but knowing my limits has been key. I follow my asthma action plan religiously and ensure my home is allergen-free. I also practice yoga and mindfulness to reduce stress."

• Q: What advice would you give to someone newly diagnosed with asthma?

• Emily: "Don't let asthma define you. Educate yourself, follow your treatment plan, and stay positive. You can lead a normal, active life with proper management."

2. Interview with Tom Martinez:

Background:

• Tom Martinez, a 40-year-old software engineer, experienced his first asthma attack during a camping trip five years ago.

• He has since learned to manage his condition while enjoying his outdoor hobbies.

Interview Excerpts:

• Q: How did you feel when you experienced your first asthma attack?

• Tom: "It was terrifying. I felt like I couldn't breathe, and I was in the middle of nowhere. After that incident, I knew I had to take my health seriously."

• Q: What changes have you made to manage your asthma?

• Tom: "I avoid known triggers like smoke and certain pollen. I also make sure to have my rescue inhaler with me at all times, especially when I'm hiking or camping. Regular check-ups with my pulmonologist have also been crucial."

• Q: What has been your biggest challenge and how did you overcome it?

• Tom: "The biggest challenge was accepting that I had to change my lifestyle. But I found new ways to enjoy my hobbies safely, like choosing less allergenic locations for camping and timing my outdoor activities when pollen counts are low."

Success Stories and Testimonials

1. Sarah's Journey to Symptom-Free Living:

• Background: Sarah, a 35-year-old mother of two, struggled with severe asthma symptoms that affected her daily life.

• Success Story: By working closely with her healthcare team, Sarah identified her triggers and adjusted her environment and diet accordingly. She also started using a combination of controller medications and alternative therapies like acupuncture. Today, Sarah reports being symptom-free for over a year and enjoys an active lifestyle with her children.

• Testimonial: "Asthma doesn't control me anymore. With the right plan and support, I've reclaimed my life. I'm grateful for the guidance and resources that helped me get here."

2. James' Athletic Achievements:

• Background: James, a 22-year-old college student and athlete, faced significant obstacles due to exercise-induced asthma.

• Success Story: Through a tailored asthma management plan that included pre-exercise medication, breathing exercises, and dietary adjustments, James was able to participate in competitive sports again. He recently completed his first triathlon.

• Testimonial: "Asthma used to hold me back, but now it's just another aspect of my training. Proper management has allowed me to pursue my athletic dreams without fear."

3. Mia's Advocacy and Awareness Efforts:

• Background: Mia, a 30-year-old environmental scientist, turned her asthma struggles into advocacy efforts.

• Success Story: After experiencing the impact of poor air quality on her asthma, Mia began working on projects aimed at improving urban air quality. Her efforts have raised awareness and led to local policy changes that benefit individuals with respiratory conditions.

• Testimonial: "Asthma gave me a purpose. I'm proud to be part of a movement that helps others breathe easier.

It's incredibly rewarding to see the positive changes we're making.

These personal stories and testimonials highlight the resilience and determination of individuals managing asthma. Their experiences offer hope and practical insights to others facing similar challenges. Through shared experiences and expert advice, the "Asthma and Diet" aims to empower readers to take control of their asthma, improve their quality of life, and achieve their goals.

CHAPTER 16

Expert Tips and Advice

Insights from Nutritionists

Nutrition plays a crucial role in managing asthma symptoms and improving overall respiratory health. Leading nutritionists share their insights and recommendations for creating an asthma-friendly diet that supports optimal lung function and reduces inflammation.

1. Dr. Rachel Adams, Registered Dietitian Nutritionist (RDN):

Key Recommendations:

• Anti-Inflammatory Foods: "Incorporating anti-inflammatory foods into your diet can significantly reduce asthma symptoms. Focus on fruits and vegetables, especially those rich in antioxidants like berries, leafy greens, and bell peppers. These foods help combat oxidative stress and inflammation in the airways."

• Omega-3 Fatty Acids: "Foods high in omega-3 fatty acids, such as salmon, flaxseeds, and walnuts, have been shown to reduce inflammation and improve lung function. Including these foods in your weekly meal plan can have a positive impact on asthma management."

Tips for Asthma-Friendly Eating:

• Colorful Plate: "Aim to fill half of your plate with a variety of colorful fruits and vegetables at each meal. This ensures you're getting a wide range of nutrients and antioxidants that support respiratory health."

• Healthy Fats: "Incorporate healthy fats from sources like avocados, nuts, seeds, and olive oil. These fats have anti-inflammatory properties and support overall health."

2. Linda Carter, Certified Nutrition Specialist (CNS):
Key Recommendations:

• Avoiding Common Triggers: "Certain foods and food additives can trigger asthma symptoms in some individuals. Common culprits include sulfites found in dried fruits and wine, as well as artificial preservatives and colorings. It's important to read food labels carefully and avoid these triggers."

• Magnesium and Vitamin D: "Magnesium and vitamin D are essential for lung function and immune health. Foods like spinach, pumpkin seeds, and fortified dairy products are excellent sources. Consider speaking with your healthcare provider about testing your vitamin D levels and possibly supplementing if needed."

Tips for Asthma-Friendly Eating:

• Balanced Meals: "Ensure your meals are balanced with a good mix of proteins, healthy fats, and carbohydrates. This helps maintain stable blood sugar levels and prevents inflammation."

• Hydration: "Staying well-hydrated is essential for keeping the airways moist and reducing the likelihood of irritation. Drink plenty of water throughout the day and include hydrating foods like cucumbers, melons, and soups in your diet."

3. Dr. Michael Roberts, PhD in Nutritional Sciences:

Key Recommendations:

• Probiotics and Gut Health: "Emerging research suggests that gut health plays a role in immune function and inflammation. Probiotics found in fermented foods like yogurt, kefir, sauerkraut, and kimchi can support a healthy gut microbiome, which in turn may help manage asthma symptoms."

• Low-Glycemic Index Foods: "Foods with a low glycemic index (GI) help maintain stable blood sugar levels, reducing systemic inflammation. Opt for whole grains, legumes, and non-starchy vegetables instead of refined grains and sugary snacks."

Tips for Asthma-Friendly Eating:

• Consistent Meal Times: "Eating at regular intervals helps prevent blood sugar spikes and dips, which can contribute to inflammation. Try to eat balanced meals and snacks at consistent times each day."

• Mindful Eating: "Practice mindful eating by paying attention to your body's hunger and fullness cues. This can help you make healthier food choices and avoid overeating, which can exacerbate asthma symptoms.

Incorporating the insights and recommendations from nutrition experts can significantly improve asthma management and overall health. By focusing on anti-inflammatory foods, healthy fats, essential nutrients, and avoiding common dietary triggers, individuals with asthma can take proactive steps towards better respiratory health. The "Asthma and Diet" provides practical tips and evidence-based strategies to help readers create a diet that supports their unique needs and enhances their quality of life.

Medical Professionals' Recommendations

The recommendations of medical professionals, including allergists, pulmonologists, and general practitioners, are essential for developing effective asthma management strategies. These experts offer valuable insights into how diet, lifestyle changes, and medical treatments can work together to manage asthma symptoms and improve quality of life.

1. Dr. Sarah Thompson, Allergist and Immunologist:

Key Recommendations:

• Personalized Asthma Action Plan: "It's crucial for every asthma patient to have a personalized asthma action plan. This plan should include details on daily medications, how to handle asthma triggers, and what to do during an asthma attack. Regular follow-ups with your healthcare provider are essential to keep the plan up-to-date."

• Avoiding Known Triggers: "Identifying and avoiding known triggers such as pollen, dust mites, pet dander, and certain foods is vital. An allergist can help determine your specific triggers through testing and monitoring."

Dietary Tips:

• Elimination Diets: "In some cases, elimination diets can help identify food-related triggers. Under medical supervision, you can gradually reintroduce foods to see if they cause any symptoms."

• Nutrient-Rich Diet: "A diet rich in antioxidants, vitamins, and minerals supports overall health and immune function. Incorporating plenty of fruits and vegetables can help reduce inflammation in the airways."

2. Dr. Michael Lee, Pulmonologist:

Key Recommendations:

• Medication Adherence: "Consistent use of prescribed controller medications, such as inhaled corticosteroids, is critical for managing chronic asthma. These medications help reduce inflammation and prevent asthma attacks."

• Peak Flow Monitoring: "Using a peak flow meter daily can help monitor lung function and detect early signs of an asthma flare-up. Keeping a diary of peak flow readings can provide valuable information for your healthcare provider."

Lifestyle Tips:

• Regular Exercise: "Engaging in regular, moderate exercise can improve lung function and overall fitness. Activities such as swimming, walking, and cycling are excellent choices for asthma patients. However, it's important to warm up properly and have your rescue inhaler on hand."

• Environmental Control: "Taking steps to control your environment, such as using air purifiers, maintaining a clean home, and avoiding exposure to tobacco smoke, can significantly reduce asthma symptoms."

3. Dr. Laura Williams, General Practitioner:

Key Recommendations:

• Comprehensive Health Management: "Asthma is often linked to other health conditions such as allergies, obesity, and GERD (gastroesophageal reflux disease). Managing these conditions through a holistic approach can improve asthma control."

• Vaccinations: "Staying up-to-date with vaccinations, particularly the flu vaccine and pneumococcal vaccine, can prevent respiratory infections that may exacerbate asthma."

Diet and Nutrition Tips:

• Balanced Diet: "A balanced diet that includes lean proteins, healthy fats, whole grains, and a variety of fruits and vegetables is essential. This supports overall health and helps maintain a healthy weight, which is beneficial for asthma management."

• Hydration: "Proper hydration is important for maintaining the health of the respiratory tract. Drinking plenty of water and including hydrating foods in your diet can help keep mucus thin and easier to clear from the lungs.

Medical professionals emphasize the importance of a comprehensive approach to asthma management, combining medication, lifestyle adjustments, and dietary changes. By adhering to a personalized asthma action plan, avoiding known triggers, and maintaining overall health through a balanced diet and regular exercise, individuals with asthma can significantly improve their quality of life. The "Asthma and Diet" incorporates these expert recommendations to provide readers with a holistic guide to managing asthma effectively.

CHAPTER 17

Summary of Key Points

The "Asthma and Diet" provides a comprehensive guide to managing asthma through dietary and lifestyle changes. Here, I summarize the key points covered in each section to reinforce the crucial strategies and information shared throughout the book.

1. Welcome to the Asthma and Diet

• Purpose and Goals: This book aims to provide practical, evidence-based dietary strategies to manage asthma symptoms and improve overall health.

• How to Use This Book: Readers are guided on how to navigate the book, utilize the meal plans, and integrate the tips into their daily lives.

• Who This Book Is For: This handbook is designed for individuals with asthma, their caregivers, and anyone interested in managing asthma through diet.

2. Understanding Asthma

• What is Asthma? An overview of asthma, its definition, and its impact on the respiratory system.

• Types of Asthma: A breakdown of various asthma types, such as allergic, non-allergic, exercise-induced, and occupational asthma.

• Common Symptoms: Identifying symptoms like wheezing, shortness of breath, chest tightness, and coughing.

Causes and Triggers of Asthma:

• Environmental Factors: Pollution, allergens, and weather conditions.

• Genetic Factors: Family history and genetic predisposition.

• Lifestyle Factors: Diet, exercise, and stress management.

3. The Role of Diet in Asthma Management

• How Diet Affects Asthma: The connection between diet and respiratory health.

• Overview of Diet and Respiratory Health: The importance of a balanced diet in supporting lung function.

• Scientific Studies and Evidence: Research findings on the impact of diet on asthma symptoms and overall health.

4. Foods That May Trigger Asthma

• Common Food Allergens: Foods like nuts, dairy, shellfish, and gluten that may trigger asthma symptoms.

• Food Additives and Preservatives: The impact of sulfites, artificial colorings, and preservatives.

• Case Studies and Examples: Real-life cases of dietary triggers affecting asthma patients.

5. Developing an Asthma-Friendly Diet

Essential Nutrients for Asthma Management:

• Vitamins and Minerals: The role of vitamin D, magnesium, and other essential nutrients.

• Antioxidants and Anti-inflammatory Compounds: Foods that reduce inflammation.

• Omega-3 Fatty Acids: The benefits of including omega-3 rich foods like fish and flaxseeds.

Foods to Include in Your Diet:

• Fruits and Vegetables: Emphasizing a variety of colorful produce.

• Lean Proteins: Sources like chicken, turkey, and legumes.

• Whole Grains and Healthy Fats: The importance of whole grains and fats from nuts, seeds, and olive oil.

Foods to Avoid:

• Processed Foods: The risks of consuming heavily processed foods.

• Sugary Drinks and Snacks: Reducing sugar intake.

• High-Sodium Foods: Avoiding foods high in salt.

6. Meal Planning and Recipes

• Creating an Asthma-Friendly Meal Plan: Tips and strategies for effective meal planning.

• Sample Weekly Meal Plans: Example meal plans to get started.

• Grocery Shopping Guide: Tips for shopping smart and avoiding trigger foods.

• Breakfast Recipes: Ideas for nutrient-rich smoothies, anti-inflammatory bowls, and whole grain options.

• Lunch Recipes: Light salads, protein-packed wraps, and asthma-friendly soups.

• Dinner Recipes: Balanced entrees, vegetable-forward dishes, and omega-3 rich meals.

• Snack and Dessert Recipes: Healthy snacks, low-sugar desserts, and anti-inflammatory snacks.

7. Lifestyle and Asthma Management

Exercise and Physical Activity:

• Benefits of Exercise for Asthma: Improving lung function and overall health.

• Recommended Activities and Precautions: Safe exercise options and precautions to take.

Stress Management:

• The Impact of Stress on Asthma: Understanding how stress affects asthma.

• Techniques for Reducing Stress: Practical strategies for stress reduction.

Environmental Factors:

• Creating an Asthma-Friendly Home: Tips for reducing indoor triggers.

• Managing Outdoor Triggers: Strategies for dealing with environmental factors outside the home.

8. Personal Stories and Expert Advice

• Real-life Stories: Sharing experiences of individuals managing asthma through diet.

• Interviews with Asthma Patients: Insights from those living with asthma.

• Success Stories and Testimonials: Inspirational stories of improved health and well-being.

Expert Tips and Advice:

• Insights from Nutritionists: Dietary recommendations for asthma management.

- Medical Professionals' Recommendations: Comprehensive health management tips from allergists, pulmonologists, and general practitioners.

By summarizing these key points, readers can quickly revisit important information and reinforce their understanding of how to manage asthma through dietary and lifestyle changes. The "Asthma and Diet" aims to empower individuals with asthma to take control of their health and enhance their quality of life through informed and practical strategies.

Encouragement and Motivation

Managing asthma can be a challenging journey, but it is one that you can take control of with the right tools and information. The "Asthma and Diet" aims to be a valuable resource in your quest for better health and well-being. Remember, every small step you take towards a healthier diet and lifestyle can have a significant impact on your asthma management.

Staying Positive and Motivated

• Celebrate Small Wins: Every improvement, no matter how small, is a victory. Celebrate your successes, whether it's finding a new favorite asthma-friendly recipe, successfully avoiding a known trigger, or noticing fewer asthma symptoms.

• Stay Informed: Knowledge is power. Continue educating yourself about asthma and the latest research on diet and health. This will empower you to make informed decisions and stay proactive in your asthma management.

• Seek Support: You are not alone on this journey. Reach out to support groups, healthcare providers, friends, and family. Sharing your experiences and learning from others can provide encouragement and new perspectives.

Embracing a Healthy Lifestyle

• Consistency is Key: Developing and maintaining healthy habits takes time. Stay consistent with your new dietary choices and lifestyle changes, and be patient with yourself. Progress may be gradual, but it is progress nonetheless.

• Mindfulness and Stress Reduction: Incorporate mindfulness practices, such as meditation, yoga, or deep breathing exercises, to reduce stress. Managing stress effectively can significantly improve your asthma symptoms and overall quality of life.

• Physical Activity: Regular exercise, tailored to your capabilities and limitations, can strengthen your respiratory system and enhance your overall health. Choose activities that you enjoy and can sustain long-term.

Next Steps for Readers: Now that you have a comprehensive understanding of how diet and lifestyle can impact asthma management, it's time to take actionable steps towards implementing these strategies in your daily life.

Creating Your Personal Action Plan

1. Set Clear Goals: Define what you want to achieve with your asthma management plan. Your goals could include reducing the frequency of asthma attacks,

minimizing medication reliance, or improving overall health and energy levels.

2. Develop a Routine: Establish a daily routine that includes asthma-friendly meals, regular exercise, stress management practices, and proper medication adherence. Consistency will help solidify these habits.

3. Monitor Your Progress: Keep a journal or use an app to track your asthma symptoms, dietary choices, exercise routines, and any changes you observe. Monitoring your progress will help you identify what works best for you.

Implementing Dietary Changes

• Start with Small Changes: Begin by incorporating more asthma-friendly foods into your diet, such as fruits, vegetables, lean proteins, and whole grains. Gradually reduce your intake of processed foods, sugary snacks, and high-sodium foods.

• Plan Your Meals: Use the sample meal plans and recipes provided in this book to plan your weekly meals. Meal planning will help you stay organized, save time, and ensure you have asthma-friendly options readily available.

• Grocery Shopping: Follow the grocery shopping guide to make informed choices while shopping. Focus on fresh, whole foods and avoid items that contain known allergens or triggers.

Engaging with Healthcare Providers

• Regular Check-Ups: Schedule regular check-ups with your healthcare provider to monitor your asthma and adjust your management plan as needed. Discuss any dietary changes and get their input on your progress.

• Seek Professional Advice: If needed, consult a nutritionist or dietitian who specializes in asthma or respiratory health. They can provide personalized guidance and help tailor your diet to meet your specific needs.

Connecting with the Community

• Join Support Groups: Look for local or online support groups for individuals with asthma. Connecting with others who share similar experiences can provide emotional support, practical tips, and a sense of community.

• Share Your Journey: Consider sharing your progress and experiences with friends, family, or on social media. Your story could inspire and motivate others who are managing asthma.

By taking these steps, you can harness the power of diet and lifestyle to manage your asthma effectively and enhance your overall quality of life. The "Asthma and Diet" is just the beginning of your journey towards better health. Stay committed, stay positive, and remember that you have the power to make a difference in your own life.

CHAPTER 18

Glossary of Terms

This glossary is designed to help you understand key terms related to asthma and nutrition that are used throughout the "Asthma and Diet." Familiarizing yourself with these terms will enhance your understanding of the information provided and assist you in effectively managing your asthma through dietary choices.

Allergen: A substance that can cause an allergic reaction. Common allergens include pollen, pet dander, and certain foods.

Anti-inflammatory: Refers to substances or foods that reduce inflammation in the body, which can help manage asthma symptoms.

Antioxidants: Compounds found in foods that can prevent or slow damage to cells caused by free radicals. Common antioxidants include vitamins C and E, beta-carotene, and selenium.

Asthma: A chronic respiratory condition characterized by airway inflammation and constriction, leading to difficulty breathing.

Beta-carotene: A red-orange pigment found in plants and fruits, especially carrots and colorful vegetables, that the body can convert into vitamin A.

Bronchodilator: A medication that relaxes the muscles around the airways, making it easier to breathe. Often used to treat asthma symptoms.

Cold Reading: A technique used in mentalism that involves making high-probability guesses and analyzing a person's responses to predict or reveal information about them.

Corticosteroids: A class of steroid hormones that are used to reduce inflammation in the body, commonly prescribed for asthma.

Cyanobacteria: A phylum of bacteria that obtain their energy through photosynthesis. They are important in the context of omega-3 fatty acids, as they are a primary source of these fats in marine food chains.

Dietary Fiber: A type of carbohydrate that the body cannot digest. Found in fruits, vegetables, whole grains, and legumes, it helps regulate the body's use of sugars.

DPI (Dry Powder Inhaler): A type of inhaler used to deliver medication to the lungs in the form of a dry powder.

Eczema: A condition that causes the skin to become itchy, red, and inflamed. Often associated with asthma and allergies.

EPA (Eicosapentaenoic Acid): An omega-3 fatty acid found in fish oil that has anti-inflammatory properties.

Flavonoids: A group of plant metabolites that have been shown to provide health benefits through cell signaling pathways and antioxidant effects.

Free Radicals: Unstable molecules that can damage cells, contributing to aging and diseases.

Gluten: A protein found in wheat, barley, and rye that can cause allergic reactions or sensitivities in some individuals.

Histamine: A compound released by cells in response to injury and in allergic and inflammatory reactions, causing contraction of smooth muscle and dilation of capillaries.

IgE (Immunoglobulin E): An antibody associated with allergic reactions.

Inflammation: A natural response of the body's immune system to injury or infection, which can become chronic in conditions like asthma.

Magnesium: A mineral involved in numerous bodily functions, including muscle and nerve function. It may help reduce asthma symptoms.

Nebulizer: A device that turns liquid medicine into a mist to be inhaled into the lungs, commonly used for asthma treatment.

Non-allergic Asthma: Asthma that is not triggered by allergens but by factors such as stress, exercise, or cold air.

Omega-3 Fatty Acids: Essential fats found in fish and some plant sources that have anti-inflammatory properties.

Oxidative Stress: An imbalance between free radicals and antioxidants in the body, which can lead to cell and tissue damage.

Palming: A sleight-of-hand technique used in magic tricks where an object is secretly held in the palm of the hand.

Peak Flow Meter: A device that measures how well air moves out of the lungs, helping to monitor asthma control.

Respiratory Health: The health and function of the lungs and respiratory system.

Rhinitis: Inflammation and swelling of the mucous membrane of the nose, often associated with allergies and asthma.

Spirometry: A common test used to assess how well your lungs work is by measuring how much air you inhale, how much you exhale, and how quickly you exhale.

Sulphites: Preservatives used in food and drinks that can trigger asthma symptoms in some people.

Triggers: Factors or substances that cause asthma symptoms to worsen, including allergens, smoke, pollution, and stress.

Vitamin D: A vitamin that helps regulate the immune system and has been linked to respiratory health.

Understanding of the terminology used in the "Asthma and Diet." Familiarizing yourself with these terms will help you better navigate the book and apply the information to your daily life for effective asthma management.

Frequently Asked Questions (FAQs)

Q1: What is the main goal of Asthma and Diet?

A: The primary goal of the Asthma and Diet is to provide comprehensive information on how dietary choices and lifestyle changes can help manage and alleviate asthma symptoms. By understanding the role of nutrition and making informed food choices, individuals with asthma can improve their overall respiratory health and quality of life.

Q2: How can diet affect asthma symptoms?

A: Diet can significantly impact asthma symptoms by influencing inflammation, immune response, and overall respiratory health. Certain foods and nutrients have anti-inflammatory properties that can help reduce airway inflammation, while others may trigger allergic reactions or exacerbate symptoms.

Q3: Are there specific foods that asthma patients should avoid?

A: Yes, some foods can trigger asthma symptoms in certain individuals. Common food allergens such as dairy, eggs, nuts, and shellfish may need to be avoided. Additionally, processed foods, sugary drinks, high-sodium foods, and food additives like sulfites can also contribute to asthma symptoms.

Q4: What foods are beneficial for asthma management?

A: Foods rich in antioxidants, anti-inflammatory compounds, vitamins, and minerals are beneficial for asthma management. These include fruits, vegetables, whole grains, lean proteins, and foods high in omega-3 fatty acids, such as fish. Including these foods in your diet can help support respiratory health and reduce inflammation.

Q5: How can I create an asthma-friendly meal plan?

A: To create an asthma-friendly meal plan, focus on incorporating a variety of nutrient-dense foods that support respiratory health. Plan meals that include plenty of fruits and vegetables, lean proteins, whole grains, and healthy fats. Avoid common triggers and allergens. Utilize the sample meal plans and recipes provided in the book for guidance.

Q6: Can exercise help with asthma management?

A: Yes, regular exercise can help improve lung function, reduce asthma symptoms, and enhance overall health. However, it's important to choose the right types of exercise and take necessary precautions. Activities like swimming, walking, and yoga are generally well-tolerated by individuals with asthma.

Q7: What role does stress play in asthma symptoms?

A: Stress can exacerbate asthma symptoms by triggering inflammation and constriction of the airways. Managing stress through techniques such as mindfulness, deep breathing exercises, and regular physical activity can help reduce the frequency and severity of asthma attacks.

Q8: How can I make my home more asthma-friendly?

A: To create an asthma-friendly home, reduce exposure to common triggers such as dust mites, pet dander, mold, and tobacco smoke. Use hypoallergenic bedding, maintain clean and well-ventilated living spaces, and consider using air purifiers. Regular cleaning and minimizing the use of strong chemicals can also help.

Q9: Is it necessary to consult a healthcare professional before making dietary changes?

A: Yes, it is advisable to consult with a healthcare professional, such as a doctor or a registered dietitian, before making significant dietary changes, especially if you have asthma. They can provide personalized advice, ensure that your dietary plan meets your nutritional needs, and monitor your asthma management.

Q10: Can children with asthma benefit from an asthma-friendly diet?

A: Absolutely. Children with asthma can benefit greatly from a diet that supports respiratory health. Ensuring they receive essential nutrients and avoiding common food triggers can help manage their symptoms and improve their overall well-being. Always consult with a pediatrician or dietitian for age-appropriate dietary recommendations.

Q11: Are there any supplements that can help with asthma management?

A: Some supplements, such as omega-3 fatty acids, vitamin D, and magnesium, have shown potential benefits for asthma management. However, it is important to consult with a healthcare professional before starting any supplements to ensure they are appropriate for your individual needs and to avoid potential interactions with medications.

Q12: Can lifestyle changes really make a difference in asthma management?

A: Yes, lifestyle changes, including a healthy diet, regular exercise, stress management, and creating an asthma-friendly environment, can significantly impact asthma management. These changes can help reduce symptoms, decrease the frequency of asthma attacks, and improve overall quality of life.

These frequently asked questions aim to address common concerns and provide clear, concise answers to help you better understand and manage asthma through dietary and lifestyle changes. For more detailed information, refer to the relevant sections within the "Asthma and Diet."

CONCLUSION

As we conclude our journey through 'Asthma and Diet', I hope you've gained valuable knowledge and practical tools to effectively manage your asthma through nutrition and lifestyle adjustments. By understanding asthma's complexities, its triggers, and the crucial role of diet in inflammation and respiratory health, you've taken significant strides towards enhancing your well-being.

This handbook has covered the impact of essential nutrients, beneficial foods, and those to avoid, as well as guidance on creating personalized meal plans, preparing healthy recipes, and making informed grocery choices. Additionally, we've explored the importance of regular exercise, stress management techniques, and creating a supportive home environment. Remember, asthma management requires ongoing attention to your body's needs and responses. By maintaining a balanced diet, staying physically active, and minimizing environmental triggers, you can reduce symptom frequency and severity, leading to improved quality of life.

I encourage you to continue exploring new ways to support your respiratory health and seek personalized guidance from healthcare professionals. With dedication and knowledge, you can achieve greater control over your asthma and enjoy a life filled with vitality and well-being.

Thank you for joining me on this journey towards better health with 'Asthma and Diet'. May you continue to breathe easier and live better, every day.